REVISED AND UPDATED

Dementia

THE ONE-STOP GUIDE

Practical advice for
families, professionals and
people living with dementia
and Alzheimer's disease

June Andrews

SOUVENIR
PRESS

This revised edition published in 2020 by Souvenir Press

First published in Great Britain in 2015 by
Profile Books Ltd
29 Cloth Fair
London
ECIA 7JQ
www.profilebooks.co.uk

10 9 8 7 6 5 4 3 2 1

Typeset in Dante by MacGuru Ltd
Printed and bound in Great Britain by
CPI Group (UK) Ltd, Croydon, CR0 4YY

A CIP catalogue record for this book is available from the British Library.

ISBN 978 1 78816 505 1
eISBN 978 1 78283 694 0

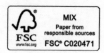

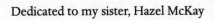
Dedicated to my sister, Hazel McKay

Contents

Preface

Dear Reader

I knew nothing really of dementia before working on the film biography of Iris Murdoch. I was delighted to have played the part of Iris and learned a great deal about this condition from others working on the project who had direct experience of Alzheimer's disease. I'm very, very pleased that if the film did anything, it put this illness in the spotlight for perhaps the first time. In the years after I undertook this role, I watched the dementia work of the Iris Murdoch Centre, which was funded by the Dementia Services Development Trust at the University of Stirling, and I have become an ambassador for those who help people with Alzheimer's disease, doing what I can to support them in raising awareness.

Dementia: The One-Stop Guide became an instant best-seller in the UK because it is so clear and practical, and I commend this second edition to you, which has been updated based on the feedback from people affected by dementia and their carers.

It was very daunting playing the role of a woman with dementia for a film, but no comparison to those who suffer with dementia or those who care for them. I hope this book will help families and friends of people with dementia, and be a support to those professionals who work to improve their difficult journey.

With love and good wishes,

Judi Dench

Introduction

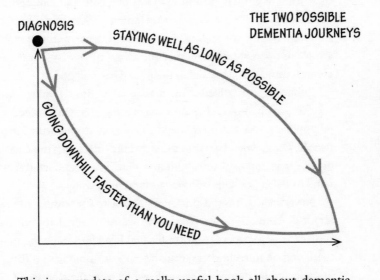

DIAGNOSIS

THE TWO POSSIBLE
DEMENTIA JOURNEYS

STAYING WELL AS LONG AS POSSIBLE

GOING DOWNHILL FASTER THAN YOU NEED

This is an update of a really useful book all about dementia
and what happens when someone is affected by it. The word
'dementia' is used to describe the collection of warning signs
that show up when your brain stops working as well as it used
to. It is defined as dementia only if these signs continue to get
worse, with a permanent deterioration over time. If you know
about dementia you will be better able to look after yourself or
someone in your family who is affected by it.

Interest in dementia in the media has never been so great.

Films have been made about famous people who had dementia. *Iris*, starring Dame Judi Dench, tells the true story of the English novelist Iris Murdoch from her brilliant youth to her last days in a care home. *The Iron Lady* is a moving film which explores Margaret Thatcher's life through fragments of history that represent her disintegrating thinking and recollection clouded by dementia (and some rather impressive hallucinations). Movies also explore ethical issues of caring. *Away from Her* and *The Savages* describe the caring dilemmas of a husband in one case and children in the other. *Still Alice* is about the rare inherited form of dementia. Although there is still stigma, this public airing means that people are more open about dementia and allow themselves to think about it more than they did in the past. This is all good.

Public figures affected by dementia in their families are recruited as champions by dementia charities and encouraged to talk publicly about dementia and share their stories with other people. Often when I get into a taxi and the driver asks me what I do, I hear a personal story about how dementia has affected their family. Once upon a time it was a shameful secret.

Nevertheless, it is still almost impossible to get sensible advice about dementia. We are faced with waves of publicity on the subject as newspapers print misleading headlines implying that there will be miracle cures available almost immediately. Families affected by dementia live in fear of losing their entire life's savings in care-home fees. Television adverts encourage us to be positive about dementia while at the same time celebrities and thought leaders say that they'd rather have cancer, or that they believe they'd have a duty to kill themselves if they had dementia. Investigative reporters make TV shows out of the misery of vulnerable people who have been on the receiving end of bad care. Scandalous nursing-home stories ruin our confidence that there might be a nursing home anywhere in which residents, even if they deteriorate, have the benefit of comfort and good cheer. The often-reported heartbreaking treatment of patients with dementia in hospital makes us afraid for ourselves and our older relatives.

In the middle of all this, thousands of people every year get the shocking news that someone in their family has dementia. For many of them their experience unfolds as if no one has ever travelled this path before. They are in uncharted territory, often surrounded by health and social care workers who don't know a huge amount about the condition. For many people it is hard to know where to turn for sensible advice.

How do I know this? In 2011, with Professor Allan House, a liaison psychiatrist, I wrote a book in plain language called *10 Helpful Hints for Carers* based on the existing research. Our printers' proof copies kept being 'borrowed' by doctors, who did not return them. When it was published, families read it avidly. Within two years over 30,000 copies had been sold, or exchanged for donations for the Dementia Services Development Trust, the charity that supported us. Families said, 'Why did no one ever tell us these things before?' Health and social care workers and volunteers took more and more copies, to give to patients, to families and to fellow workers who had never been taught about dementia in their training. At last there was some sensible and practical advice for anyone trying to make things better for people with dementia. But it was not enough. *Dementia: The One-Stop Guide* was written to give more information and advice about how to cope with the dementia journey the best way you can.

Everyone has a unique experience, but in general there are two possible routes with dementia. On one track you stay as well as possible for as long as possible, living life the way you want to. On the other you go downhill faster than you need to, for reasons that are often avoidable. Everyone would like to avoid unnecessary trouble and expense, and to delay some of the difficult situations that might arise. Sensible, practical advice on how to do this is in short supply. People aren't told about the remarkable services and equipment that are readily available or the simple changes to their lifestyle that can be so radical that they prevent the need to go into a care home.

Dementia: The One-Stop Guide provides detailed information about what will make a difference in the lives of people with dementia and their carers. It is practical and compact, and builds on the *10 Helpful Hints*. Some information is repeated in different chapters, to save the reader from having to flip back and forwards. In setting out to write this, I've drawn on information that is freely available if you've got a clinical qualification that prepares you to understand it and a few months to research it. However, when someone in your family gets dementia you may not have that sort of time. This book is for you.

Chapter 1

What is dementia?

People use the term dementia to mean a number of things. This chapter will give you a basic understanding of the commonest types of dementia and why it is useful to know the difference between them for practical reasons. Dementia is much more than just a memory problem and you might find that some of the professionals you meet are misinformed about it, so the more you know the better.

A range of diseases can cause the changes in the brain that give rise to dementia symptoms. There are probably more than a hundred of these diseases, but three or four of them are very common. The commonest is Alzheimer's disease. Up until recently, student doctors and nurses were told little if anything about dementia. And if they were told anything, it was often wrong. They were told not to worry about what underlying ailment was causing the patient to have the dementia signs and symptoms. This way of thinking was known by real experts to be wrong long before it was ever corrected in the education of the professionals. People were misinformed. It was lazy thinking, which was inexcusable, even though there was not enough research on the subject.

What did they used to say in the past? In my own experience I've heard all of these misleading statements ... and there are more:

● It's just a memory problem.

● We shouldn't worry patients about this because we can't be sure of the diagnosis.

● You can't really tell for sure what disease is causing the problem until the post-mortem, so that limits what you can do for them.

● There is no point in raising the question of an underlying disease with the patient or their family because there is nothing that can be done.

● The treatment is the same no matter what the cause, so even the doctors and nurses don't need to distinguish between the possible causes of dementia.

● It's part of normal ageing – you expect and accept these symptoms in old people.

● It's a wasting disease – you can expect them to lose weight and die quite quickly.

In the course of this chapter I'll show that all of these assertions are wrong, but you need to be aware that this is what was taught to very many of the doctors, nurses, social workers and others you might meet. You'll end up knowing more than they do. But you have to work with these people, so how you handle that difference in your level of knowledge can be tricky. The situation is getting better with all the recent public interest in dementia, but research shows that even if the professionals who are now working in the health and social care system received any dementia education in their undergraduate or pre-registration training, it was more likely to be about the anatomy and physiology of the declining brain tissue than about answers to practical questions, like what you should do if the person starts getting lost in the night. I hesitate to say that it was useless, but certainly the education has not been good enough from the point of view of carers or people with dementia who come to professionals looking for help. Most of the people with dementia seen by students in the past were in hospital and largely unable to do even the most basic tasks, and often they were behaving in very disturbing ways. That's how medical people viewed dementia – they expected dramatic and painful debilitation and chaos. They never realised that 75 per cent of people with dementia were living quietly at home.

Things are a bit better now. There is a lot of publicity and more education. All the people who have been formally diagnosed with dementia are listed on a register at their GP's surgery, so that they can be considered for help, treatment and support. (At least they should be … in some cases the clinic doing the diagnosis fails to communicate it to the GP.) Their carer is given a right to support through this mechanism. The Health Departments in the UK provide an incentive to family doctors by giving them an extra payment for putting people on the register. So that's good. What's more, many people are getting their diagnosis (if they get a diagnosis) at earlier stages of the condition, when they still have a lot of independence and can enjoy life, exercising their capacity to make decisions and have fun. That early diagnosis also means that they have more potential benefit from the limited range of medication that is available and can plan their future better.

But when you ask the question 'Is this dementia?' you are still dependent on a doctor to put a name to the troubling symptoms that have beset you or your loved one. If the doctor remembers his or her training and it was as bad as mine was, they'll not feel confident enough to make a diagnosis, and might still believe there is no point in trying. This means that you might have to push for that diagnosis. There is huge variation across the UK. At the time of writing the first edition of this book in 2015, in Scotland and Northern Ireland two-thirds to three-quarters of the people with dementia symptoms had been given a diagnosis. In some parts of England as few as 20 per cent of the people with dementia symptoms had their diagnosis. In total on average across all of England they were missing more than half of people at the time. The situation has improved, but even so there is a widening gap between what people with dementia should expect to receive as care, and what is available for them.

Particularly when they are older or if someone in their family has had dementia, people worry about whether they themselves are getting dementia. It's all over the news, and in surveys the majority of respondents say they'd rather have cancer, so it is clearly terrifying. Sometimes people who think they have it try to hide it. Couples collude with each other, pretending that everything is all right when it isn't. Children worry about their parents and may be fearful of raising the subject. Friends don't like to mention it in case they cause offence. That's understandable, but there is no justification for any doctors to still actively avoid addressing the issue, though they clearly do.

What can you – as families and patients – do, given all the rules about patient confidentiality, if you have difficulty getting a GP to take your concerns seriously? The first step is to find out for yourself as much as you can about dementia and the associated problems. That will give you power.

Things that look like dementia but aren't
Mild cognitive impairment
There is a condition called mild cognitive impairment (MCI), which many of us will get if we are lucky enough to grow old. Because some people who get dementia start with MCI it can be very worrying to have it. But cheer up! Studies show that the majority of individuals with this memory loss never progress to

having full-blown dementia, and MCI itself can sometimes be reversed or at least remain stable. You need to know what to do about MCI and how not to worry, but you also need to be sure to see a doctor if you really think it is progressing to become dementia.

If you have MCI you may have minor difficulties with memory and attention, and some language issues. It is like being mentally tired all the time. In fact it can be brought on by stress and fatigue, or another illness, but unlike dementia it is potentially reversible and not necessarily progressive.

People with MCI have problems that are less extreme than people with dementia. At least 5 per cent of older people have MCI, depending on how you define it. It would be really useful if you could tell which of those are going to go on to develop dementia, but at present there is no real way of knowing, so that means there is a limit to what doctors can do. There is limited evidence that brain exercises might help, and all the things that you will read about later in this book that help reduce dementia symptoms are probably sensible to consider as a precaution in MCI.

Delirium

Another condition, called delirium, is a fluctuating temporary confusion that often happens to older people when they are ill because of something else, such as a urine infection, or too many pills, or a chest infection. Delirium can be dangerous if it is not treated and people die as a result. Sometimes it is an early sign that the person is likely to get dementia in years to come, so if you've had it your GP needs to be told. If delirium occurs in hospital, it may not get treated if staff see the older person in bed being 'confused' and don't think there is anything abnormal with that. As is made clear in Chapter 12, you need to make sure medical and nursing staff know if the level of confusion is a change and a deterioration from how the person usually is and you need to persuade the doctors and nurses to treat the cause.

Depression

In addition, if an older person gets depression, that may look a lot like dementia. Fortunately, depression can be treated and reversed. It is tragic if the health care staff wrongly assume that it is dementia and that nothing can be done (because they are then wrong on two counts, as both dementia and depression can be helped). Carers need to be on their toes to make sure that unintended harm does not occur either because some doctors don't diagnose delirium or depression or dementia, or because they try but their diagnosis is wrong.

What are the symptoms of dementia?

The key symptoms of dementia include:

- difficulty in remembering things;
- difficulty in working things out;
- difficulty in learning anything new;
- difficulty in coping with any physical or sensory impairments that develop as a result of normal ageing or the result of illness or accidents;
- difficulty in finding your way about and driving.

These symptoms don't come alone. There will be other issues, depending on what the underlying disease process is, and different symptoms come to the fore at different times. People with dementia often have language problems and their behaviour may change. The key problem is a reduction in the person's capacity to do everything. Put together, these symptoms cause phenomenal stress and a crushing fatigue. So it is really important to take the symptoms seriously, even in the very early stages.

I went to the doctor to say I was having problems with calculations, and he laughed and said that I was still better at maths than him. I assumed he was just reassuring me with a little pleasantry and that he'd refer me to a specialist but he did nothing. (Retired scientist, 78)

Remembering things

Memory is not the worst for me. I've learned to use a lot of props – diaries, Post-it notes, electronic things like my ... What's it called? ... hand phone ... mobile ... What was I saying? ... [prompted: 'Forgetting?'] Yes ... People think I've forgotten how to do things ... but it's as if time has gone funny. I stare at the task for ages and then realise that ten minutes have passed and I've not done it ... [long pause] ... I've not forgotten how to do it. I just somehow forget to start ... and then I'm slow. (Early-retired nurse, 57)

There is no doubt that people with dementia have memory problems. When they lose memories of past events, it often happens in a characteristic way where the most recent memories fade fastest. People may describe a situation in which they can recall the names of all the members of all the pop groups from thirty years ago, but they're not sure if they ate lunch today. They may remember how to use skills that they learned in childhood or early adulthood, but more recently learned things are slipping away from them.

One way this shows up is people going home to the wrong house – maybe the house they lived in twenty years ago. They don't 'remember' where they now live. Another distressing example is failing to recognise close family members.

Every single time I see my uncle he looks at me as if he is puzzled and says, 'You've changed. You look different.' Even if he saw me only the day before … I've realised now that his memory of me is fixed about fifteen or twenty years ago, before my hair and beard started to go grey. He recognises me, but within twenty-four hours he's forgotten again that I'm in my fifties and he's still expecting the thirty-something me when I knock on his door the next morning. (Nephew, 55)

This can be really painful for family members, particularly young ones. As recent additions to the family tree, they are the first to disappear from the story. When you think of the excitement and joy of the birth of a grandchild, and the special relationship with a grandparent, it is almost unbearable that they may one day look at the child or young person and say, 'And who are you, young lady?' You need to think about how you are going to explain this when children ask, 'Does Granny not love me any more? Why doesn't she know me?' There are books which explore these issues sensitively with young people and internationally a number of children's authors set out stories about this in beautifully illustrated and carefully crafted books that you may feel comfortable reading with smaller children (see Resources and helpful organisations, page 320). When someone makes a mistake like this, they feel embarrassment and shame, or confusion and anger – a whole range of emotions – so think about how to handle conversations in a way that helps to keep things calm. Maintaining a tranquil atmosphere makes a huge difference if you can manage it.

It is even more crushing if your mother or father stops knowing who you are. You arrive at the house and start to bring in the shopping for them and they shout at you and tell you to go away. 'If you don't leave at once I'll get my son to deal with you,' your mother says. 'But I *am* your son!'

People do really believe that in some sense their mother

has died if she does not know them any more and that they are meeting a stranger who inhabits their mother's body. One strategy to try is to ask your mother if she has a daughter or son, and see her face light up as she tells you all about her darling, then remember that, in truth, that's you.

There are no rules about how to handle this. A key message is that the person with dementia has worse symptoms if they are facing a lot of challenges. See if you can avoid unnecessary challenges. And there are lots of things that can help with memory difficulties at different stages of the dementia. There is more about this later in the book.

You should see our fridge. It is covered with magnets holding notes up for Mum reminding her about stuff. I know that she studies the notes and uses them. I've passed the kitchen door and glanced in to see her with her glasses on the end of her nose, peering at them. (Daughter, 57)

Working things out

Difficulty in working things out is sometimes described as 'loss of executive function'. Not being able to remember things becomes a serious issue if you are unable to undertake this basic function, which normally compensates for memory gaps in most people. Imagine waking up in a hospital bed. It may take a few moments to work out where you are and what to do. There are lots of clues – machines and people in uniforms, and curtains and lockers. You don't remember how you got there, but you've worked out where you are so there are possible explanations. Did I have an accident? If the nurse comes and tells you that you were knocked off your bike and hit your head, and that you'll be fine and your son has rung from work and is on his way to the hospital, then you can relax on your pillows and think, Wow, that was a lucky escape.

Now again imagine waking up not knowing where you are. Nothing round you gives you a clue. There are machines and people in uniforms, and curtains and lockers that remind you of … what? You can't think. The nurse comes and tells you why you are there, and seconds later you can't remember her or what she said. You decide to get up and explore and you can't work out where you are. The more you struggle to understand the less sense it makes. You start to wonder if you've been drugged and brought here against your will. Then panic sets in as you realise that your young son must be waiting for you at the school gate. You need to leave. Someone tries to stop you and you fight them and they sedate you.

Both patients have a memory problem. They can't remember how they got to where they are. One can work it out, and make use of new information presented to him, but the other can't and dredges up old or invented bits of information to try to fill the gaps. The first situation becomes more reassuring by the minute, while the second becomes more nightmarish. That's what dementia feels like. It's intensely stressful.

Where am I? Where am I? I am in hell. (Plea from a woman with dementia in an acute hospital, quoted by a hospital visitor.)

There are very many activities we do every day on autopilot, but if you break them down they are really complicated executive functions. Just getting out to work, even if you have no family responsibilities, is complex. You need to be organised the night before, and have clean appropriate clothes ready to put on, and in the morning you need to get out of your nightclothes, eat, shower and shave or put on make-up and check your home is secure, before heading off with your travel ticket or car keys. If you have lost executive function you may know you have to do these things, but not be able to put it all together. A lady found in the street in her nightclothes has not necessarily 'forgotten' to get dressed. She's just not putting things together as she did every day of her life till now. Because of difficulties in thinking, she is in fact preparing for a day in the past. She's long retired. She has nowhere she needs to go, no matter how overwhelming her sense that she must get up and get on with things. And so she left the house before dressing or eating. Insight into how loss of the capacity to work things out and loss of executive function disable people with dementia gives us a clue about how to handle this sort of situation. You can avoid a lot of trouble if you try very hard to get inside the head of the person with dementia. Not trying is the mistake that many professionals make. This lady does not need to be 'put away for her own safety'. She more probably needs some prompting and distracting at the time of day that she is most likely to set off on the wrong track, and that may be not random but the same time every day, making it easy for you to work out how to resolve the problem.

Learning anything new

Being aware of the difficulty with new learning is vital for under-standing and managing the problem that people with dementia have of forgetting recent things. When we are children and our brains are developing our parents and teachers rehearse us over and over until knowledge 'sinks in'. Every toddler who learns when asked 'What does the dog say?' to reply 'Bow-wow!' knows they will be rewarded with laughter and attention. Training humans and other animals to respond to a reward is well recognised as a deliberate teaching technique and we use it instinctively with babies. This is a form of 'operant conditioning', which is a process where behaviour is modified by the consequence of the behaviour. It's an important part of learning. You do something again because of the positive outcome. But what happens if you can't make the connection between what you did and what happened next?

A very small number of children develop a form of dementia. A good understanding of the limitations of traditional teaching methods is really important for those who are caring for them. Because they are at school, they are in an environment where people are rewarded for new learning, and where teachers go over things again and again until pupils know them. When the child starts to say he does not know what he knew yesterday, he may be suspected of being lazy or wilfully naughty. Parents even get angry and frustrated. The particular children who have the disorders that can be seen as 'dementia' have mostly started life with a learning difficulty in any case, so the disintegration of what they have achieved with so much effort is a double tragedy. Their families have to learn quickly how to cope with this new reality and stop 'rewarding' 'good' behaviour and 'discouraging' the 'wrong' behaviour. What works with other kids is just frustrating and confusing for children with dementia. In caring for adults with dementia we have a great deal to learn from these resourceful families, teachers and paediatricians who are managing a reduction in the capacity to learn in this very small group of children.

Not least, we all need to learn from the children that when we point out that something has not been learned by the person with dementia they will feel shame and anger with themselves. Given that we ought to know that they have problems learning, why would we be so insensitive?

In the hospital ward, I was talking to the consultant and we were interrupted by the presence of an old man who was clearly busting to ask a question. He was neatly dressed, washed and shaved and very polite. 'Doctor, I'm ready to go now. When am I going home?' The doctor sighed and all but rolled his eyes and said, 'I told you already that will be Friday.' I've never seen such a crestfallen look on anyone's face. The patient wasn't just disappointed, but profoundly embarrassed to discover that he'd already been annoying the Great Man with his stupid questions. He looked slapped. Almost immediately he could not remember the exchange but his sense of discomfort lasted much longer than the memory of how he'd gone wrong. He retained a profound reduction in his self-confidence. (Hospital visitor)

Because the person has difficulty with learning new things, it is as if they have forgotten. When the nurse says, 'But I told her where the toilet is and how to use the call button,' she is displaying a lack of understanding. The person with dementia may have forgotten these instructions before the nurse has finished reciting them. They never learned them at the time. We have to ask ourselves why we want this person to learn a new thing, such as how to get the nurse by pressing the button or that they should not press the button every thirty seconds. If reaching a nurse when you need one depends on you learning a new skill under current hospital arrangements, we need to change the hospital arrangements. When up to 50 per cent of hospitalised patients have confusion, why would you equip the staff with a complex, unfamiliar method for their patients to call for help? The person with dementia in these circumstances may find it beyond them to learn to use it properly. It's not impossible to learn new things after diagnosis, but in general this capacity is starting to slip and it will continue to do so over time. It's bizarre that a nurse would describe someone as 'forgetting' something they never learned.

Coping with physical or sensory impairments

Mother had apparently said to the nurses, 'I can't read.' So when the mobile library went round they just passed her by. Actually she loves to read, and I got her a bright light and some large-print books, and she devoured them. They said to me, 'We actually thought she was not able to read. We did not realise.' They thought it was the dementia. I'm saddened by their ignorance and confusion about dementia because it is her that suffers when THEY get confused. (Daughter of Mary, 85)

It is important to remember that about 5 per cent of people with dementia are of working age. That used to be forgotten. The other 95 per cent are old or very old. All older people will experience the changes of ageing, which usually include physical or sensory impairment. Reading glasses, walking aids and hearing aids are getting less expensive and more sophisticated all the time, so most of us are compensating well. However, if you have a problem with learning new things, you may be unable to use some of the aids that are available. It could be as simple as not remembering to put on your glasses, or failing to eat properly because you have forgotten how to use your dentures.

The loss of confidence that follows as a result of adverse incidents created by these problems can lead to someone not wanting to go out and about any more. The person with dementia has even greater difficulty in adapting to changes in their physical capacity than other older people. For example, if you aren't good at remembering where you are, it is really important for you to be able to see where you are. All older people need more light because of age-related changes in the eye, but if you've got dementia it matters even more. The increased light will help you to see objects you might have forgotten, and gives more information to help you work things out. (See Chapter 9 for ideas on lighting design.) But if you have dementia you may forget to put the light on, or make an unwise decision to economise on the electricity, not realising how false that economy would be.

In addition, depending on what the underlying cause of the dementia is, you might have other problems. For example, people with vascular dementia are more likely to have spatial-awareness problems that create a risk that they will fall over. Fear of falling is very debilitating for older people. If they have already fallen and suffered a fracture, the patient with dementia in hospital may not remember that they mustn't try to stand alone while they are undergoing rehabilitation. There is a great temptation under these circumstances to use restraints, like safety straps that tie them to a chair. But in the end this may cause even more injury as the person tries to escape, having forgotten (or never learned) why they are tied down.

I will never use restraints again, or allow my nurses to use them. I wish I could get them banned altogether. I walked on to the ward one day just as one of the patients had wriggled and wriggled in her seat to try to get out, and she had slipped down and the lap strap was at her throat. Everyone was busy and had not noticed. If I had not walked by at that moment she would have been strangled. (Ward sister)

Finding your way about and driving

People with dementia are sometimes described as 'wandering'. Some objections have been raised to using that term because it implies that the person is drifting around for no reason and that they are lost. Curiously, the person is not lost, but rather looking in a determined and rational way for something which unfortunately is no longer there, or trying to enter a building that no longer belongs to them.

Our neighbour moved away a short distance, and after she often came striding along our street staring at each door in turn. We'd go out to meet her, and distract her with conversation and gossip while walking her round the corner to her daughter's house. She kept wandering back to our street, though. (Neighbour)

It is useful to consider what underlies this problem. Dementia robs people of their most recent memories, so they may forget that they moved to a new house.

Driving is made hazardous for similar reasons. When you learn to drive you pick up some really important skills, such as how to use a roundabout. If you were to travel as the crow flies, you'd go round anticlockwise to turn right, rather than driving all the way round and taking the last exit. The person with dementia who decides to take the short route is being perfectly logical, but has forgotten the rules of the road and the danger of ignoring them. Turning right into a dual carriageway is more complicated than you think. If you've tried to drive in a country where the rules of the road are different, you will know how challenging that is.

Driving demands quick judgement and adherence to certain rules, and the person with dementia is slowed in their judgement and has forgotten some of the rules. This is why you are legally required to tell the DVLA that you have been diagnosed with dementia. Failure to do so will incur penalties, but people are so disabled by losing their car that they are tempted to avoid revealing their news.

In the end we had to take the car away from the house, so even Mum could not use it. While it was there, Dad used to threaten her to get the keys, and drive off. He was so angry. When he first was diagnosed he had a driving test and they let him drive for quite a while after that, but eventually he failed the test. It is really hard, but I'd rather that he was angry with us than that we were explaining to someone why he had run over their child at a crossing point. (Son of Roger, 79)

In some countries you can get a provisional licence that allows you to drive in a restricted area, as long as someone is with you in the vehicle. It may be frustrating to go back to being like a learner, but in reality, with dementia, you become more 'inexperienced' as a driver with the passage of time as the recent memories and skills fade.

Stress

All five of the symptoms outlined here (remembering, working things out, learning, coping and finding your way) give rise to dreadful stress. It is stress that explains some of the dementia-related disturbing behaviour that families and professionals find hard to understand. The more challenging the environment is for people with dementia, the more stress they will suffer. The main challenges have been identified by research. They include the behaviour of other people, the hazards in the physical environment in terms of noise and light, and the design of spaces. Another challenge is presented when the person is required to go through rapid change and faces too many people and new systems and processes. The person may already be undermined physically by poor diet, lack of exercise and even dehydration, on top of whatever cocktail of medicines they have to take for their other ailments. Any intervention that can be made to reduce stress will certainly make life easier, both for the person with dementia and for the carer.

What are the different diseases that can cause these symptoms?

Alzheimer's disease

Alzheimer's disease has long been considered the most common cause of dementia and about half a million people in the UK are affected by it. Seen through a microscope, abnormal clumps appear in the brain tissue, along with tangled fibres that should not be there. There is a loss of connection between brain cells, which eventually die. It is clear that the brain damage starts long before there are any behaviour symptoms. A person might not have ever had dementia symptoms in their lifetime, but might be found to have those changes in the brain tissue caused by Alzheimer's disease at a post-mortem examination. As an affected person gets older, more brain cells die and whole regions of the brain start to shrink so unmistakably that you can see it on simple brain scans. The cause of the disease is not fully understood and that hampers attempts to find a possible cure. It mainly affects old or very old people, and the older you are the more likely you are to be affected.

It seems that people who have the Alzheimer's disease changes in their brains, but no dementia symptoms, have some form of resilience. This could be because of lifestyle things like exercise and not smoking, or having learned another language, having avoided some common conditions like depression that seem to make dementia more likely, or simply because of luck. We just don't know. But it makes it hard to find a medicine to prevent this sort of dementia, because you don't even know which of the people with Alzheimer's brain changes will get the dementia. Thus you wouldn't be able to tell whether a dementia medicine worked, because the person may not have been about to get dementia anyway.

Of course families wonder if it is inherited. The position is complicated. Families who have a record of living to a great age include lots of relatives who lived long enough to get dementia.

Well, the doctor says I'm getting the dementia now and I am celebrating. I'm ninety-six, you know, and I did not die in an accident or from cancer or in the war, and I've still most of my teeth (enough anyway) and something has to get you in the end. It's OK. All my brothers and sisters lived to be over ninety and I was the youngest. It's just my time. Two of them had it, but not bad. (Retired schoolteacher)

Researchers look at what we now call the 'Fourth Age'. This term is used to classify people over eighty-five. They are extreme survivors. It is as if those of us under that age are still being 'weeded out', but if you make it to eighty-five you may be around for much longer and are probably really tough in a way that is worth studying.

If you are unfortunate enough to be in a family where anyone got Alzheimer's disease before they were sixty years old, then your family is possibly affected by a dementia that has more inherited factors than the others. One explanation for the lack of knowledge about family connections in the past was the stigma that used to surround any mental health problem. Someone with 'early-onset' or 'working-age' dementia these days will sometimes reveal that one of their parents did die young, but no one ever talked to them about the cause of death, and it was swept under the carpet so they didn't know much about it as children, and now no one is alive who knew. Many people in these families will never get dementia, though, and it is important to ask your GP for genetic counselling if worry about this is affecting your life.

Would you take a test to find out if you'll ever develop dementia? After seeing both her grandfather and father succumb to the disease, 35-year-old Hannah Mackay made the decision to take the test. Not only was she given the tragic news that she'll develop dementia within the next twenty years, but that her two young daughters also have a 50 per cent chance of inheriting the disease.

Refusing to accept this 'death sentence', police-sergeant Hannah is now focused on enjoying her life to its fullest, and raising awareness in the hope of finding a cure. (ITV This Morning; 17 July 2019)

This heroic young mother took the test, she told me, because she knows that her daughters may have the same inherited condition, and she wants to show them that a person can live a good life and a happy one, even if they know that there are very serious problems ahead. The film *Still Alice* has a moving fictional account of the struggles of a family where one child inherits the gene from Alice, one does not, and a third just does not want to know. There is evidence that lifestyle changes can delay the onset of symptoms even in these cases, even though the outcome cannot be escaped. But it is to be remembered that they are very rare.

In Alzheimer's disease the causes of the plaques and tangles are still to be worked out. The amount of time and money spent on Alzheimer's disease research has increased in recent years. Dementia is so expensive to society and so feared that there will be great prizes and financial rewards for anyone who can find a cure for even just the Alzheimer type. Cruelly, there are press stories nearly every week about the latest breakthrough, but on closer reading they are usually unconvincing. The increases in research money announced in the UK are from a very low level – only a fraction of what is spent on cancer research. This is ironic when you realise that dementia costs more than cancer, heart disease and stroke put together. Around £23 billion was spent on managing dementia in 2012 in the UK.

The research spending more than doubled in the next three years, but it was still only a small fraction of what was spent on cancer research. The total spent on medical research during this time was measured at about £31.4 billion and only about 2 per cent was spent on dementia. Although a number of charities give some money for dementia research, the only dedicated research charity is Alzheimer's Research UK. A new dementia research institute has been set up in the UK through the Medical Research Council. But there is a long way to go. Drug companies in 2019 have been abandoning their attempts to find a medicine for Alzheimer's, because their lack of success so far has made it financially impossible to keep trying.

A number of years ago when it was reported in the newspapers that there were high levels of aluminium in abnormal Alzheimer's disease brain tissue, people threw out all their metal pots and pans and bought glass ones. That was pointless, because we get aluminium in our diet anyway from a range of other sources, including indigestion remedies, but it illustrates how people react to single 'research discovery' stories in the news. It is ironic that the evidence that exercise makes a difference has been building up all the time, but you don't really see that coming through on health education messages. We don't see people throwing away their sofa to avoid memory loss … but all of us ought to be sitting down less.

The important thing to remember about Alzheimer's disease is that it's a gradual process that starts years before any symptoms set in. So if you know someone has Alzheimer's disease and their dementia symptoms suddenly become very much worse, it is unlikely that the Alzheimer's disease process is causing this sudden deterioration. It's more likely that they've got some other illness brewing, like an infection or a delirium. If they are treated, the person can go back towards their previous level of functioning. Knowing the diagnosis also allows the person or their carers to take particular care when the person gets other illnesses.

This retired teacher with Alzheimer's disease was living well at home in the house she had occupied for fifty years, just having daily visits from the daughter. She was discovered fallen one day and taken to hospital, where she was diagnosed with a urinary tract infection and started on antibiotics, but unfortunately she had a fall while in hospital when she confused the location of the toilet and fractured her hip. Rehabilitation was slow and she became disturbed and was judged unfit to return home, having failed a kitchen assessment with the OT staff. Care home destination was recommended. In the care home she was agitated and aggressive and antipsychotic medication was prescribed, and shortly after this she had a stroke and died. It is my view that if the urinary tract infection had been treated at home this lady would be alive today. We could have tried harder. (Specialist dementia nurse)

In Alzheimer's disease it is particularly valuable to have an early diagnosis because there is some Alzheimer's-specific medication that can help, and you can't access that till you've been diagnosed. Also, it works best in the early stages, so you don't want to miss that window of opportunity. There are lifestyle changes that you can make to significantly reduce the symptoms, even though they don't alter the disease process a lot. They are worthwhile because they make the journey easier, and some of them are enjoyable in their own right, but the medication is time-sensitive.

The organisations in each country of the world which support people with dementia and their carers are almost universally known as 'Alzheimer's' organisations, a convention that has sprung up because in many languages the word 'dementia' has offensive connotations. Although called 'Alzheimer's', they take an interest in other non-Alzheimer's types of dementia, and want to influence policies that will affect all causes of dementia. Those organisations, supported by overarching organisations like Alzheimer's Disease International (ADI) and Alzheimer's Europe, have played an important part in raising political awareness of dementia. One of the most helpful tools in their work is the increasing amount of evidence about the financial cost of dementia to society, and their prediction that numbers affected are going to double in the next twenty years. In any country it may be that the finance minister has as much interest in this as the health minister. This is why the UK government chose dementia as its theme for a G8 summit in 2013 and every year more countries launch a dementia strategy.

There are a couple of good reasons for emphasising the linguistic point. When the media gets excited about 'developments in treatment' or 'cures' for 'Alzheimer's disease' (or 'AD') it is important to question whether they really mean Alzheimer's, or if they are referring to all forms of dementia. The truth is that even if we did have a way of preventing Alzheimer's disease today a lot of other people would still develop dementia symptoms, because they had been harbouring the disease for decades or because their particular dementia was not caused by Alzheimer's. And the search for the cure for other causes of dementia would still need to go on.

LATE

In recent times a 'new' form of dementia has been discovered. The name doesn't trip off the tongue: limbic-predominant age-related TDP-43 encephalopathy. It is known as LATE for short. There is stuff accumulating in the brain just like in Alzheimer's, but it is a different type of protein. It is said that up to a third of people diagnosed with Alzheimer's may have LATE instead, or they might have a mixture. It has been suggested that up till now Alzheimer's treatments have seemed to fail because the new drug was clearing up the Alzheimer's disease, but LATE was developing at the same time, and remaining unaffected. So the dementia stayed, caused first by AD and then by LATE. This is an important discovery for research, but understanding is still at the earliest stage and it doesn't make much practical difference currently.

Vascular disease

This is the next most common cause of dementia, affecting about 20 per cent of people with a diagnosis of dementia. The problem here is the blood supply to the brain. The symptoms generally come on more suddenly than in Alzheimer's disease. It may happen after a stroke or a series of strokes. What makes vascular dementia like a stroke is that both are caused by disruption to the brain's blood supply, as a result of which a bit of brain tissue dies. It can be caused by burst blood vessels or blood clots blocking vessels. The Australian dementia organisations coined a great phrase: 'What's good for your heart is good for your head.' Any health problems that are likely to cause difficulties with blood circulation and increase the risk of heart attack will increase the risk of vascular dementia. This would include high blood pressure, diabetes, high cholesterol and any heart-related problems – and in addition all the lifestyle issues that make those conditions worse, like lack of exercise, smoking and eating too much of the wrong sort of food.

One of the biggest differences between vascular dementia and Alzheimer's dementia lies in the underlying disease process. In Alzheimer's or LATE the brain shrinks relatively slowly as individual brain cells die back and so the symptoms creep up over time. In vascular dementia there is a distinct moment when the blood vessel gets blocked or bursts. The person can be stable for a long period and then deteriorate suddenly to a lower level of functioning as another bunch of blood vessels get damaged. Blockage is more likely when there is narrowing of the blood vessel caused by thickening of the wall where fat deposits have gathered. The symptoms of vascular dementia depend on which part of the brain has been damaged. The commonest form is called 'multi-infarct' dementia. This is where there are lots of tiny strokes taking out lots of different areas. Each lobe of the brain does a different job and doctors can tell where the damage was from scans. That knowledge can give some insight into what problems you might expect. Deep inside the brain, at what is called the 'subcortical' level, there are tiny blood vessels which can be damaged when the person has a stroke. This is called sub-cortical vascular dementia or sometimes Binswanger's disease. The symptoms of that dementia include difficulties in walking, clumsiness, lack of facial expression and speech difficulties. About 10 per cent of people with dementia have a mixture of vascular disease and Alzheimer's.

My dad had a small stroke and then declined rapidly over twelve months, and he's in a home now after his second stroke, but I met a man who told me he has vascular dementia as well and he's living at home. His experience was that he got very bad over a few months and since then he's been stable for three years. It seems that everyone is different. (Son of man with multi-infarct dementia, 72)

Vascular dementia can run in a family if the family has a history of stroke or cardiovascular disease. Indian, Pakistani, African-Caribbean and Sri Lankan communities have a high prevalence of vascular risk factors and more research needs to be done to see how their risk can be reduced. Vascular dementia is progressive, but treating the underlying medical conditions can help to slow the rate of decline. This includes managing the high blood pressure, cholesterol, diabetes or heart problems. There is no recommended drug for the vascular dementia itself, unlike Alzheimer's disease, but if the patient has a mixed dementia the Alzheimer's medication may be recommended. However, given the recent emphasis on public health measures like smoking bans and education about keeping fit, it is interesting that this coin-cides with an unpredicted downward trend in the prevalence of dementia. It is too soon to say that this means we're preventing it, but that would be the logical conclusion. And wonderful, if true.

How many people die with dementia? The publicity currently says that it's the second leading cause of death, and that's an interesting number. The WHO (World Health Organization) says between 5 and 8 per cent of the population aged sixty and over have it. It depends what the UK Office for National Statistics means when they say it 'accounts for 12.7 per cent of all deaths'. Is it just a question of what takes you in the end? I can't get my head round it. (Journalist)

Neither can I! You may as well say they are dying of austerity because the mortality rate seems to depend on the services. (Professor J Andrews)

Dementia with Lewy bodies (Lewy body dementia)

Lewy bodies are tiny lumps of protein in the brain which disrupt normal functioning. No one really knows where they come from or how they do this. Similar abnormal proteins are found also in the brains of people with Parkinson's disease. Unfortunately many people with Parkinson's do go on to develop dementia that resembles the Lewy body type of dementia.

About one in ten people with dementia have this type. It is rare below sixty-five years of age, but not unknown. Because it is rare it is not always spotted and gets mistaken for Alzheimer's disease. The person may get some symptoms of Parkinson's disease, which include loss of facial expression, an inclination to shuffle and limb stiffness. People describe vivid hallucinations.

Dad was kind of rooted in his chair and I was trying to get him to mobilise a bit. I thought the problem was the muscle stiffness, but he said that he was afraid if he stood up he might hurt the little animals that were sitting on the carpet round his chair. (Daughter of Mr B., 67)

In Chapter 8 there is more discussion about what you can do when someone is hallucinating. These symptoms ebb and flow on a daily or hourly basis. It is not unusual for the person to doze a lot during the day and then have agitated nights troubled by hallucinations and nightmares. They will have falls and fainting attacks. That combination of fluctuation and hallucinations is what will lead the doctor to think that it is the Lewy body type of dementia.

Lewy body disease is the prime example of why it is useful to know what the underlying cause of the dementia is. It is not unusual for a person with dementia to exhibit disturbing behaviour. It is regrettably not unusual for them to be prescribed antipsychotic medication in a rather slapdash approach as an attempt to tranquillise them.

The message here is that antipsychotics should only be used in very specific circumstances in order to treat psychotic symptoms and never used just for the sedative effect (which is often called a 'chemical restraint'). By 'psychotic' symptoms I mean delusions and hallucinations which are so disturbing for the patient that you really need to do something to help them. If you prescribe them at all it should be done with extreme caution in dementia with Lewy bodies and Parkinson's disease. I'm tempted almost to say 'never' in Lewy body disease. (Dr Cesar Rodriguez, Consultant Old Age Psychiatrist)

Even where there are no serious side effects, this medication often does not work and yet it continues to be administered despite the fact that it is extremely dangerous and can cause strokes or other fatal complications. But in Lewy body dementia specifically there is a particular risk from antipsychotics that will reduce life expectancy and cause very disturbing side effects that are irreversible if you don't catch them early.

Our aunt was admitted to a care home where they told me she was 'resistive to care', whatever that means, and they put her on some medication and she just stopped. I mean she stopped walking, and eating. She lay on her bed and was as stiff as a board. It was like she was dying. [A friend] ... recommended that I ask them for a list of her medication and they refused that day, but the next day they gave me one. I did not understand but it was very short. They said they'd had the doctor in and he had reduced some stuff. She started to get better almost at once. She is her old self. (Nephew of retired schoolteacher, 80)

It appears that by asking the question about medication this family had alerted the staff and prompted them to get it checked, even though the family didn't understand the list when it came. Perhaps the doctor stopped the antipsychotic medicine when it was drawn to his attention that someone was checking. You can always check out a list of medications with a pharmacist – the community pharmacist at your local chemist shop. They are smart and they love to look for medicines that you shouldn't take because of something else you have wrong with you and medicines that don't mix well. It is called 'deprescribing' and it's highly recommended by geriatricians. Your pharmacist is your friend. A list of the names of some of those dangerous medicines might help, but names change and the same medicine can have more than one name. This is because each company that produces it can give its own product a name in addition to the general name, which is called the 'proprietary' name.*

The drugs for Alzheimer's are not 'licensed' for use in patients

---

* At the time of writing, these antipsychotics had names like aripiprazole (Abilify), chlorpromazine (Largactil), clopenthixol (Clopixol), haloperidol (Haldol, Serenace), olanzapine (Zyprexa), promazinequetiapine (Seroquel), risperidone (Risperdal), sulpiride (Dolmatil, Sulparex, Sulpitil), trifluoperazine (Stelazine). It is worth checking.

with Lewy body dementia, but they are sometimes used with good effect. Licensing a drug means approving it formally for a particular type of patient. In using them outside of the licence, the doctor is taking a calculated risk in the belief that it will benefit the patient.

My husband was in hospital and I took him out every day, usually home or doing our usual things, but I could not cope at night. He had to go back. He had "night terrors" which were nightmares that made it dangerous to be around him. I've had more than one black eye. (Wife of Fred, with Lewy Body Dementia)

Frontotemporal dementia

This is the name given to a range of conditions including Pick's disease and the dementia that comes with motor neurone disease. These conditions are grouped together because the part of the brain affected in each case is the area responsible for behaviour, emotions and language, and so the problems that the person has may be similar in each case. The brain gets a build-up of abnormal proteins, as seen in Alzheimer's disease, so that brain cells are progressively lost and the affected area of the brain shrinks. It only affects about 5% of people with dementia, so it's hard for some people to understand.

In the days when we had double rooms there was a family that asked for their grandmother to be moved out because she had started to use some really quite choice foul language. They thought she was picking it up from the other lady. It was quite a delicate job explaining that it was the dementia. As the front lobe of her brain was damaged all the proper manners and inhibitions that she had as a proper lady were breaking down, and it wasn't anyone's fault, but the disease. (Care home manager)

Although this is the tale of an older person, frontotemporal dementia is a greater cause of dementia in those under the age of sixty-five, where it is the second most common cause after early-onset Alzheimer's disease. ("Early-onset", or "young-onset" are two expressions they use when someone of "working age" gets dementia and journalists often mix that up with "early stage" dementia which just means the first signs and symptoms.) Almost half of cases have a family history of the disease, so there has been some progress in identifying the relevant genes that are causing the problems. Genes act as chemical instructions inside cells, which allow the body to make things, and if they go wrong that gives rise to problems. Some of those problems can be passed down in families because you inherit your genes from your parents, but in the other cases it is not known what causes this frontotemporal dementia. The person's behaviour and their personality alter for the worse, which is very distressing for families as the person lacks insight and loses the capacity to identify with others. They appear to become self-centred and insensitive and they may even fall foul of the law. Because the patients are younger, facilities and services are less likely to be geared up for their needs and so having an accurate diagnosis goes some way towards giving a family a strategy for living with this problem.

People think of my husband as being a rather difficult, nasty rude person, which he never ever was before. He loses his temper and annoys other people. Our children can't bring their friends to the house because he says inappropriate things. (Wife of man with frontotemporal dementia)

No one knows better what this is like than those family members who are living with it. In correspondence with me one husband has sent his own tips on "Managing the Rage Stage" and "Tips for Communicating" which we've put on the website at www.

juneandrews.net. He's not only caring for his wife but helping others to find their way. It's a real problem when you are affected by a rare and difficult form of dementia, when other people just see difficult behaviour and have no idea how to respond.

The top tips about dementia knowledge and awareness

- Be aware that a lot of the people you meet in professional jobs don't have an in-depth understanding of dementia.
- With Alzheimer's dementia there is some medication available to temporarily delay the disease processes, but otherwise treatment is all about symptom control and keeping well.
- You can find out a great deal about the sort of dementia that is affecting you or your family, but first you need a diagnosis.

Chapter 2

Getting a diagnosis

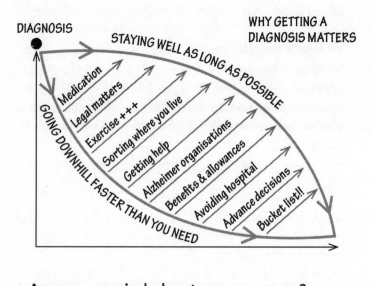

DIAGNOSIS

WHY GETTING A
DIAGNOSIS MATTERS

STAYING WELL AS LONG AS POSSIBLE

Medication

Legal matters

Exercise +++

Sorting where you live

Getting help

Alzheimer organisations

Benefits & allowances

Avoiding hospital

Advance decisions

Bucket list!!

GOING DOWNHILL FASTER THAN YOU NEED

Are you worried about your memory?

People worry about whether or not they have dementia yet avoid trying to find out. It is vital to get a diagnosis – especially because there are some conditions that look like dementia which respond really well to treatment. Facing the problem is the first step towards getting help. This chapter looks at how hard it can be to get a diagnosis and how to help someone (or yourself) through that process. The most important message to give people is that it is never too soon to see your doctor if you are worried that you might have dementia and equally it is never too late. So when should you worry?

I wish there was some advice on how to raise the issue with someone? And how to support them through the trauma of a memory test? We never asked my mother, which means that seven years on, the one person who has had no input into decisions about her care ... is Mum. And I really don't think we are unusual. (Ruth, whose mother was affected by dementia)

Ordinary forgetting

All of us forget stuff from time to time. Some people habitually forget names or are always losing bits of paper or keys. The important words here are 'habitually' and 'always'. Even though you have always been scatterbrained, you may become self-conscious about it only when you are older. You might worry that others will comment on it. How you do at maths, or map-reading, may get worse as you get older. The time to worry about dementia is when you start to get very much worse. What your family and friends notice is important, so ask them. Did I used to get mixed up like this? With luck, they'll laugh and give you funny examples from your past. You are not getting worse. That is just ordinary forgetting. There is also an element of slowing down. The older you get the more answers you will know in the pub quiz, but the younger ones will get their answers out faster than you. That's annoying and so a good reason for having a mix of ages in the team.

Dementia is not ordinary forgetting. It is ordinary to forget phone numbers. It is more worrying if you start to forget how to use a phone or what it is for. Dementia is when you have a marked reduction in your capacity to both remember and do things. If you were great at maths or map-reading you may slow down, but you should still be able to do it. If maths just doesn't make sense any more and you are holding the map upside-down or getting cross and throwing it away, it is worth thinking about seeing someone.

There is no such thing as 'normal' memory. Everyone is different. The most important concern is if you've had a progressive downhill change from what is 'normal' for you. Some people advise that you should have reached the stage where it is causing real problems in your life before thinking it might be dementia. The difficulty with this is that what causes a problem for you actually depends more on your resources than the severity of the symptoms.

Dad was reluctant to drive after he got lost a couple of times and had some scrapes trying to park and so we got him an account with a local taxi firm and he is fine now. (Daughter of 75-year-old man)

Getting your dad a chauffeur service stops the driving problem, but in case the driving problem was a sign that something major was going wrong it is worth getting him to check it out. The doctor would want to know if he's having other problems, like difficulty in following conversations, or trouble performing other familiar tasks, like changing the discs in his DVD player that he learned to use perfectly in the last few years, or managing the ATM cash-point machine.

Eleanor rammed her bus pass into the ATM to try to get cash out. When I went to speak to the bank counter staff they pointed out icily that this was the fourth or fifth time it had happened over the last two months. (Sister of retired shopworker)

If you are a member of the family and you are asked by someone if you think they're affected, don't make light of it if you yourself have concerns. Be practical and down to earth.

My brother said that he worried about his memory, so we went for a walk and talked about it together. I asked him what was happening. He described how he'd been driving home recently and found himself parking outside the old house where we used to live. He was always going upstairs to get something and by the time he got there he couldn't remember what he was going for. I pointed out to him that he'd asked me a couple of times recently for money he thought I was due to give him which I thought I'd already given. He was mortified and so was I. I had been too embarrassed to say something at the time. I tried to make him laugh by pretending to complain how he never forgets giving me money but only forgets when I've given it back. Then seriously I suggested that we go and talk to the GP about it. I went with him. (N., 68)

If you are worried it is a good idea to talk to someone who knows you well to see if they have noticed a change. They might be too embarrassed to say, so even if they give you reassurance it is best to see the doctor anyway. Write down the concerns you have. A diary is useful to help give a clear picture. It also helps you get a picture for yourself about what is happening.

Is it really dementia?

Some people don't want to raise dementia with their GP because they are afraid. They think that there is nothing to be done. They think that if it is bad news they just don't want to know. To be honest, it is always better if you go for the check-up. Some of the symptoms that look like dementia are reversible. It could be that you are coming down with something else, like depression or an infection. Because these are easily treated, it would be a mistake not to see about them and get back to normal as soon as possible. Don't just think it's your age.

He's a work colleague and we are together a lot and I've known him for years. The other day when I was telling someone about him I could not remember his name. I'd been saying how good he was and recommending him and I'm sure the other person thought I was talking rubbish. How could you recommend someone if you don't even know them well enough to remember their name? How true were the stories about our successful joint projects in the light of that? I used to be great at this. Now I find myself going round in circles. It's been for the last six months. (Professor, 58)

There is a long list of things that can affect your memory that are NOT dementia:

- loss, such as the death of someone, a divorce or job loss;
- nervous tension or worry;
- noise or other distractions;
- general medicines, particularly if you are taking more than four;
- overuse of alcohol;
- poor health;
- sadness and depression;
- side effects of sleeping pills or other sedatives;
- sleep deprivation;
- some infections, particularly in older people (chest infections and urine infections are notorious);
- the menopause;
- thyroid disorders;
- too many things on your mind;
- vitamin B12 deficiency.

Ordinary forgetting can arise for any of these reasons. Are you stressed and tired? Could you be depressed? Some women find that the hormone changes of the menopause cause psychological difficulties as well as physiological ones. Have you just got too many things to worry about?

However, if it really is dementia then spotting it at the earliest stage is a huge advantage. There is medication that can help in some cases, and you can start to put strategies in place that will let you live a happy life at home for as long as possible.

What should you do?

You should start with your GP, but don't assume you'll be heard at first. Even though the government has been saying for years that early diagnosis is really important, in some parts of the UK you've got a much lower chance of being diagnosed. If you don't get a diagnosis you don't have an explanation for the difficulties you are experiencing. It also excludes you from being offered medication, or accessing any of the supports that are outlined in this book. Research shows that some GPs dismiss anxieties until it is too late to undertake some of the really helpful interventions. What should you say to your GP to get his or her attention? What should you do if he or she seems not to be listening?

I took this daughter to see the GP who had failed to diagnose the dementia in her mother for two years, even though everyone in the family and the old lady were quite sure that something was up. I showed him all the local services that were in place that would have helped and the calculation of how many benefits this family had missed out on as a result of her not getting a diagnosis. Over the two years they were nearly £16,000 worse off. He was shocked and pointed out he did not have access to this sort of information, and I told him he only needed to remember one fact: the phone number of the local

Age UK office, where people were waiting to help families with these sorts of problems. No one was trying to attack him and we've still got a good professional relationship. He tells his colleagues. But I don't have time to visit every GP in the land. (Age UK manager)

Even so, there are many GPs who are interested and motivated to discuss this issue with you. Ask them for a double appointment because you'll be doing a lot of talking and listening. The national guideline about dementia (from an organisation called NICE, the National Institute for Health and Care Excellence, which covers England and Wales only but provides guidance similar to that in the rest of the UK) says that people worried about dementia in themselves or someone they know should be able to discuss their concerns and the option of seeking a diagnosis with someone who has knowledge and expertise. In your GP practice there may be a specialist nurse or psychologist who does this on behalf of all the GP partners. That is always a good option in my experience. They are specialists themselves and might have even more time for you. You need to take time and get information so that you can make an informed decision about what you are going to do next.

In this area we've got a clinic run by a specialist nurse called Eddie. The GPs can ask patients to make an appointment with him and he'll see them either at the surgery or in their own homes. Eddie says it is actually better in the house. (Alzheimer's Society adviser)

Local authorities and the organisations they work with, and NHS and social care staff should know about the local dementia guidelines and also how to put you in touch with someone knowledgeable with whom you can have this sort of discussion. It might be that before going to the GP you already had a chat with someone else, like a voluntary group or the manager of another service, like a care home, where the person who might have dementia is living. But it is the GP (or that specialist nurse) who is the gatekeeper for further diagnostic services in most cases.

People from black and minority ethnic groups in the UK sometimes have difficulty in getting access to good health care. This problem sometimes seems to be even worse if dementia care is needed. If you come from a culture that has a different view of dementia from the mainstream health and social services, it will be hard to get the help you need. This is an issue that needs to be addressed. There are estimated to be about 25,000 people with dementia in minority ethnic communities in the UK, and about two-thirds of them are in the London area. Carers in different communities have different views about whether services should be culturally specific or mixed. There are some very successful groups for specific national communities. In general mainstream services, people from black and minority ethnic backgrounds are so few that they are clearly not accessing the services. From the statistics we know they exist, but they are missing out on help. In a system where users have to 'fit in' they have a double jeopardy. It's hard to fit in with the mainstream system that may not be culturally sensitive to you and, in any case, people with dementia find it hard to fit in at the best of times.

What happens at the doctor's?

GPs often do a short mental test in their consulting room. They are sometimes so focused on getting the outcome they don't realise that it can be humiliating to 'fail' the test.

Mum refused to answer. It was as if the test had been designed for her to fail and she would not put herself in that position. (Daughter of 86-year-old woman)

In addition to doing a basic dementia test by asking some questions, the GP will focus on your general health. You can see a GP being interviewed about this at www.dementiatrust.org.uk/projects/wnttad/topics/gettinga-diagnosis/ Because there are so many reversible physical conditions that might be causing your problem, the GP will probably recommend blood tests to check:

- vitamin B12 and folates;
- thyroid function;
- minerals, like potassium and calcium;
- glucose;
- liver and kidneys functions;
- other routine elements, like counting the blood cells, checking for inflammation.

You might be asked for a urine specimen to see if you've got an infection in your bladder. Older people are different from younger people when they have a urine infection. Younger people complain about itching and burning and needing to run to the toilet. Older people sometimes just start to seem confused. (The hazard is if health workers assume that all old people are expected to be confused and don't test for and tackle the underlying infection that's causing it.) You might be sent for a chest X-ray if it looks like you've got a chest infection, or for a heart trace (ECG) to see if there is a problem there.

The GP, if he or she thinks it could be dementia, will send you to a memory assessment service or memory clinic, which can be provided by specialists at the hospital or from a community mental health team. This is called a 'referral'. (See Chapter 11 on what you can expect from the health care system.) You will be attending 'psychiatric' clinics. Part of the problem of asking for help for many people is the stigma about psychiatry and suspicion of those who provide psychiatric services. Don't be put off if you are sent to see someone with 'psychiatry' in their job title. You need to bite the bullet. Memory assessment services come under a variety of names but they specialise in the diagnosis and initial management of dementia and are intended to be the single point of referral for people with a possible diagnosis of dementia.

The local GP or social work professionals that you meet ought to know and understand the process of making referrals. The GP might decide that you've not got a problem that needs to be taken to the specialist clinic right now but that it would make sense to see you again in a while to assess how you are getting on and if things are becoming worse. If you think your concerns are being dismissed, you can ask to see another GP.

What should happen at the memory assessment service or memory clinic?

Then Mum went to the memory clinic. The day was very long and boring for her, and she did not like it much. But my friend has told me it depends what doctor you get. She and her mum saw a really nice one. And for them a lot of the tests were actually done at home. (Daughter of 86-year-old woman)

There is more about clinics in Chapter 11, but basically you will be asked (or should be) if you want to know the diagnosis once they have made it and who you want to share it with. Usually the assessment will include:

- 'taking a history' – that is, asking you all about what has made you go to your doctor with your current problems;
- 'cognitive and mental state examination' – that is, a test to see how well your brain is working;

- physical examination (that's what doctors do!);
- review of medication – that is, seeing if it is your pills that are causing the problem.

It's recommended that if you might have dementia but it is mild and they are not quite sure, they do further 'formal neuropsychological testing'. This means more sets of tests that are used to diagnose brain deficits and usually this will involve a one-to-one conversation in an office. There is a wide range of tests that can be used, but they focus on the areas of memory, orientation, language and problem solving.

... the consultant's conversation with Mum (who is American-born and still has her accent):
Consultant: Well, I detect that you might have a bit of an American accent. Can you tell me who is the president of the United States?
Mum: (looking blank) No, I don't think I can remember that.
Consultant: (in a desperate attempt to tap into Mum's longer-term memory) Can you remember which president was assassinated?
Mum: No, I don't.
Consultant: (by now desperately trying to give clues) He had Irish connections.
Mum: (face lighting up with sudden enlightenment) Oh, you mean O'BAMA!
(story from on-line forum)

At the time they'll also want to check if you have other medical or psychiatric problems in the picture that are making your dementia worse. It's not unusual for people diagnosed with dementia to be depressed and everyone needs to keep an eye out for that, because it can be treated. Some people claim that antidepressant medication does not work with people with dementia any more than giving them a bit of support and being sensitive to their feelings. And the last risk you need is any unnecessary pills.

As highlighted in Chapter 1, where different sorts of dementia were described, it is very important to know what 'subtype' of dementia you have: that is, which disease is causing your symptoms. This differentiation is best done by specialist staff using evidence-based criteria. It is relatively unusual for them to ask for examination of your spinal fluid, which they do through a lumbar puncture, or spinal tap, but it may happen if you volunteer to take part in research. Sometimes if it is suspected that you have a rapidly progressing form of dementia such as CJD (Creutzfeldt-Jakob disease) or that you might have another disease that can be treated, they will be able to tell that from spinal fluid drained off with a lumbar puncture. In general, EEGs (electroencephalographs or brain traces) are not used for diagnosis but might be considered when there have been epileptic fits, which sometimes come with certain sorts of dementia. They also might recommend a brain trace if there is suspected delirium, frontotemporal dementia or CJD.

MRI (magnetic resonance imaging) and CT (computerised tomography) brain scans are used to help early diagnosis and to detect subcortical changes in blood vessels (the Binswanger's sort of dementia, where blood vessels deep in the brain have been affected). These scans give good views of the underlying structure and anatomy of the brain. If the person had a previous learning disability the interpretation of these scans is difficult, but earlier diagnosis is getting better all the time.

… this time last year he was getting almost perfect scores on the tests – even though it was very obvious that he did indeed have dementia. As the consultant said, intellectual starting point and educational level can manipulate the test scores a lot. (Wife)

What if it is dementia?

At the clinic someone should take time to discuss the diagnosis with the patient and their family (if the patient agrees). It's recommended that written information is provided on the following:

- signs and symptoms;
- the course of the disease and what to expect in the future;
- treatments that are available if any;
- local care and support services;
- support groups;
- how to stay well;
- sources of financial advice;
- legal advice and advocacy;
- medico-legal issues, such as driving;
- local information resources.

Staff want to see if there are any interventions they can use that will help your cognitive symptoms (remembering, working things out ... all the mental functions) and keep you functioning at the best possible level. What is offered by the clinic, or the NHS, or social services, or local and voluntary organisations, varies all over the UK.

What they could offer will be either pharmacological or non-pharmacological.

- **Pharmacological** – that is, drugs. In terms of medicines there are two pathways. If you've been diagnosed with Alzheimer's disease there are some drugs that can be offered. The drugs available are called acetylcholinesterase inhibitors. In vascular dementia you may be offered Memantine (even though it is not licensed for such use).

● **Non-pharmacological** – that is, support and advice on lifestyle changes and everything else.

They may also offer support for psychological problems such as depression and anxiety, both of which are understandable in the circumstances, and this could be either medicines or some behaviour therapies. Everyone should be offered post-diagnostic support.

In addition the clinic can offer support for other symptoms, which are called 'non-cognitive' and include hallucinations, delusions, anxiety, agitation and aggressive behaviour. Another expression that is used is 'behaviour that challenges' or 'disturbing behaviour' and this includes wandering, agitation, hoarding, sexual disinhibition, apathy and disruptive vocal activity (which basically means shouting out). Chapter 8 is devoted to disturbing behaviour and there it is made clear that much of such behaviour is an expression of distress.

We should assume the behaviour of a person has meaning even when we find it difficult to understand. What we might regard as difficult behaviour may in fact be a logical expression of fear, anger or frustration or the pain of the person with dementia. (Managing Disturbing Behaviour, dementia.stir.ac.uk)

What really happens?

We were the last appointment of the day. The doctor asked us to wait outside for a bit. Then he came out and told us that my wife had dementia. I went home in a complete daze. He gave us nothing ... not even a leaflet. We couldn't speak to each other. We didn't know what to say. (Couple in their 70s)

People with dementia can miss out on getting a diagnosis by the proper pathway. Your GP might be one of those who don't recognise the value of a diagnosis. Your local memory assessment service may be so busy that the GP does not bother to refer you because he thinks you will wait too long and achieve nothing of value.

We were trying to convince the GPs at their group practice meeting to make more diagnoses. I pointed out that this health centre ought to have forty or fifty more people on their register according to the statistics for the local older population. I even reminded them that they would get money from the government for doing it through something called QOF [quality and outcomes framework] points. One young doctor got really incensed. 'Even for money I will not do this,' he said indignantly. 'There is no benefit to my patient in going through these tests. There's no treatment for them.' Sir Galahad, it turned out, had no idea about the twenty-four-hour helpline, the befriending service, the financial support from the local authority and, to be honest, the human right of the patient to access information about themselves. For him 'treatment' means 'prescriptions'. (Dementia diagnosis project leader)

It might be that you get a second chance of being given a diagnosis if you have to go to hospital for something else. All hospitals are supposed to check you for cognitive problems when you are admitted, particularly if you are older and appear confused. In some cases, although the check is done and the staff 'know' you've got dementia, it does not get written in your discharge letter so the GP does not 'know' and neither the GP nor the hospital refers your case to the memory assessment service. That's not good.

The person with dementia may be in a care home before someone actually puts a name to the problem.

Our mum was living at home by herself and me and my sister were taking good care of her. My sister works days in an office and I'm a van driver on nights, so we could always pop in at different times – shopping, little jobs, just a cuppa. She had a fall and she was in hospital. We wanted her home. When she did get back they said she'd have to go to a clinic. We didn't really know what it was about because we just took her there and waited for her. It was called Outpatients B. She went back and forward a few times. Then she had another fall and broke her hip. We all decided she'd be better in a nice care home, and she went to one to try it out and they said they couldn't have her because she had 'dementia'. No one had ever told us that for the two years we'd been taking her back and forward. If I'd have known maybe I could have done more and stopped her falling. No one told us what to do. No one told us nothing. (Son, aged 56, of his 75-year-old mother)

Of course, the process of getting a diagnosis is not always bad, but knowing some of the pitfalls will help you negotiate the symptoms.

I was very confused and anxious and my GP really listened to me. Of course when I got to the memory clinic and it turned out to be dementia I was devastated, but I can't fault the wonderful staff who have supported me every step of the way. I want them to know now how grateful I am that they are there for me. I'm determined to stay well for as long as possible. My friends are all around me, including the nurses and doctors. (Enid, 65)

And what if you don't have dementia ...

Well, that is a reason to be cheerful, surely, as long as you and your doctor have got to the bottom of whatever was making you worried. Get that infection treated, or sort that vitamin problem, or deal with that stress and get out of there!

It might be that they've decided you have mild cognitive impairment, which generally affects older people and means that, although you can function very well, your mental strength is declining faster than in the majority of people. One major difference from 'real' dementia is that in about half of the people affected it never gets really bad or descends into dementia. Of course it is a nuisance, but if you follow the advice in this book about keeping well, and even use some of the techniques and technology described here, you'll still be able to get on with your life as you wish and perhaps reverse those symptoms.

To stay well with MCI you may decide to adopt the same lifestyle changes that are known to help delay symptoms in people who really do have dementia. You want to keep your brain in the best shape possible, so think about the following:

- Keep up all your normal activities as much as you can for as long as you can.

- Learn a new language with a group of other people.

- Keep your mind active. There is no single preferred activity, so the one that you enjoy most will be the best because you are more likely to stick at it.

- Keep involved with family and friends and enjoy community life through your usual activities, like going to church or meeting friends in the pub ... whatever is usual for you.

- Plan ahead for situations that might become tricky, like dealing with banks and insurance (this includes arranging a power of attorney now, while you are well, for someone you trust to take care of decisions if the time should come when you are not up to it: see Chapter 13 for advice on legal issues).

- Get your medications checked regularly. The rule of thumb is that if you are on more than four it's possible that you are taking too many. The pharmacist can help check this out for you.

- Keep an eye on your blood pressure and cholesterol levels. Diet is really important for you now.
- Exercise, exercise, exercise ... This is so important. You don't have to power round the gym, just make sure you keep moving.
- Stop smoking. Now. Immediately. No arguments. If your brain is struggling it needs more fuel. The fuel it likes is oxygen. Would you put petrol in a diesel engine knowing that it would be fatally damaging? You don't want to write off your brain, do you?
- The story is similar with alcohol. You need to preserve brain cells, not destroy them. The good news is that a glass of wine a day is said to be a good thing. But if one is never enough for you it is better to have none at all.
- Reduce stress however you can and get enough sleep.

Is it rude to suggest someone has dementia?

Because I'm known as a dementia expert, people are always asking me about dementia. Even at family gatherings or parties, people will come up and say, 'Do you think I've got it?' or 'Will I get it?' I find this openness hard to match with the reluctance that people have to raise such questions with each other. I've promised my own family that if they do show signs I'll tell them. This is because the medicine only works at the early phases and I don't want them to miss out. But I know that others do not raise the matter with relatives because it might seem insulting or frightening to suggest that they appear to be failing in some way.

If you are worried about being too direct, you could try supporting a local Alzheimer's charity fund-raiser and taking your relative to the part where they do an information talk. That will help you to open the conversation, especially if the speaker is giving the message that earlier is better for diagnosis. Talk about your own fears about the possibility of ever having dementia and describe what you'd do if you ever thought you had it, then ask them what they'd do.

It might be that you just have to take the bull by the horns. You can appeal to the desire that many older people have not to be a nuisance. Overcome the stigma and taboo that you carry inside. Do your homework and make sure that you yourself see signs that are more than normal forgetting. Then be strong, as you would with any friend or family member at risk.

I said to her, 'Mother, there is so much about dementia in the news and I'm terrified that you might get it but miss out on all the medication and other help, so you MUST come with me and see about it. I insist. I'll come with you. If you are OK that's fine, but if not you'll cause us so much trouble later if you don't help us by dealing with it now. And it's not about you being forgetful, because we all have that. I just want to be sure you get tested.' (Daughter of Shakira, 79)

If the process during which the doctors ask the questions is annoying, be as supportive as you can. Most of what doctors have ever done to us is annoying, but we put up with it because they are wonderful and save our lives, or at least make them better. At this stage of life we can't do much about the stigma of 'failing' an exam, so until the doctors get more subtle in their testing techniques, make for home straight afterwards and be comforted in any way you can.

Getting a diagnosis of dementia can be a shattering experience. It is terrible luck, and everyone will be sad and upset for you. But then they must gather round you and make life the best it can possibly be … and this book will give you ideas for how that can be done.

Chapter 3

Adjusting to the news: for carers

I've learned that people will forget what you said, people will forget what you did, but people never forget how you made them feel. (Maya Angelou)

When someone close to you is diagnosed with dementia the effect can be devastating. It is the responsibility of the doctor to tell the patient, and it should be done face to face at a special appointment so that the patient can ask questions. They should have someone with them and this may be you. This is a pivotal day in your lives. It is important to get as many facts as possible, so try to take notes or ask for some written information. If the doctor is not using language you understand, interrupt them to ask questions. They might use jargon or technical terms and it is essential to ask about what they mean – they won't mind. The doctor might not try to cover every stage of the illness in the first meeting, but you should not leave without some idea of what the next step is. If you arrive home and discover that you missed the next step, you can get back in touch and ask when the time is right for you.

Remember that technically the doctor must have the consent of the person with dementia before imparting personal information to you. That consent is implied by the person taking you to the consultation, so there should be no difficulty in you taking part in the conversation. Sometimes doctors are overly cautious about confidentiality, so be prepared to make a case. In Scotland, for example, carers' rights to be part of these conversations are enshrined in law. If the person you care for can't make a decision about their health care without your help, you should be involved in decisions. You have the right to ask for a second opinion from another doctor if you are unhappy with the decision that the health professional has made. In other places, carers always need to have a power of attorney (see Chapter 13) before they are allowed to be so involved.

Of course it is bad news that someone has such a serious condition, but there is an increasing awareness that the actual process of breaking the news will significantly affect how the person is going to live from then on. This can mean different things to different people. You and the patient might be pleased to have a name to put to what is wrong.

I thought I was going mad. I thought people were breaking into my house and stealing money. Now I know it is dementia, I'm not happy about it but it is less frightening. (Retired civil servant, 78)

The information that is being given may adversely affect the person's view of their future, with the prospect of limited choices and threats to dignity and independence. However, it can actually in some cases, when done well, start a positive process of living well and extracting the best from the rest of life. Reluctance to give bad news has always been an issue in health care and doctors in the past have felt they had the right to withhold information. Doctors used to avoid telling people that they had cancer, even when it was clear that this must be the case because of the obvious treatments. What else do you get radiotherapy for? Sometimes they even withheld this information at the request of families.

Dad told me that Uncle Bill didn't want Auntie Sarah to know she had cancer. I was a young nurse at the time and I thought it was awful. We all knew, why not her? So I worked out a way of being alone with her and asked her if she wanted me to talk about her treatment. She gave me a smile and said, 'It's all right, darling. I know all I need to know.' There they were keeping their secrets and I know she knew perfectly well. It was them that needed to avoid facing it, not her. (Nurse)

It has been made clear to professionals in their guidelines that they must respect the right of the patient to know any bad news, while using professional judgement about how and when to give the full picture. Dementia care will remain far behind in achieving this standard while we still have clinicians who can't or won't address the issues.

What can you do to help?

Just by being there you have made a very good start. Not everyone has someone who cares about them at this time. You will feel anxious and devastated yourself and that needs to be dealt with, but later. This is not about you. If you are not able to be calm, you'll not be in a position to help.

When the doctor told us that Mum had dementia our world seemed to fall apart. She was so young. It was so unfair. But I had to be strong for her. I knew that the first couple of days would be the worst. She needed more information so that she could start to plan for the future. (Daughter of Ethel, 61)

When you come out of the consultation just calmly say what you are going to do next.

I got her in the car and drove her along to the abbey, and we sat on a bench near the lake. We've been there hundreds of times and I know she loves it. I had a flask of coffee with me. I must have known we were going to need it. We hardly spoke. (Husband of Ethel, 61)

You can't assume that you know what is most devastating about the news for the person concerned. It might be that her worst pain is the knowledge that she won't see her grandchildren get married, or that she's not going to be able to retire to the seaside as she always planned. Don't try to hurry anything. This dementia thing can go on for years and this is just the first day. She may have years of good health ahead of her, but this is not the time to talk about that. You are both reeling from a blow. At some point you will have to think about how and when you are going to tell other people about it all, but perhaps not yet.

Right now you are filled with care and compassion for the other person, but it's important not to be a hero. You may have to bear the brunt of anger and grief, in addition to dealing with the problems that have arisen as a result of the illness, which might include questions about future finances, car driving and how to just live together. So you need to find out how to care for yourself.

Everyone responds to these challenges in different ways. I am in awe of the carers I meet and how they manage. Here are some of the negative aspects of caring, with ideas of how to deal with them if you are affected.

Denial is a coping mechanism. It gives you time to adjust, but you can't stay like that for ever. At some point the carer has to start looking at the practical implications of what is happening and get the information that is needed to work out a plan for the future. But that doesn't happen in the first stage.

Anger is understandable. Your frustration and concern about how unfair this is may build up so much that you want to express them, but you need to find a place where it is safe to do so. In the heat of the moment it is possible to say things that you will later regret. You may have worked hard all your life, looking forward to a leisurely retirement, which now looks like being stolen. Of course you are angry.

Grief will arise from the sorrow you feel for what the other person is losing, and what you are losing yourself. To begin with you will have difficulty in thinking about anything else. You may lose yourself in sleep and then wake the next morning to feel it flooding in again. You need rest and distraction from it. This intense feeling, which is natural, will become less painful with time.

Thinking positively is a major challenge. Some of your negative thoughts are entirely rational, but you can focus on the problems too much. Live in the moment and try not to worry about the future or dwell on the past. Don't undervalue yourself and the wonderful work you are doing as a carer. Take consolation from your religion or faith. Take comfort from friends and family.

Resilience is the ability to recover from setbacks. You still feel the anger, grief and pain, but you can keep functioning. To do this you need to take care of yourself and not be afraid to ask others to help take care of you. Your resilience may be knocked, but you can recover.

Social isolation does happen when dementia strikes. It is really important to understand that friends are not a luxury; they are a necessity for maintaining your health and sanity. You need friends in order to be happy and you may need to tell them overtly that you need them. If you give them specific jobs to do for you it will help them know what you need from them.

Anxiety about the future is a common problem for carers at the time of diagnosis. The best antidote to this is to get as much information as you can about what support is available to you and what common problems you might face. You can get help and advice from Age UK, the Alzheimer's Society or any of a range of organisations listed at the end of this book.

Some carers do get affected by depression, exhaustion, sleeplessness, irritability and health problems, but many do not.

I joined the Alzheimer's carers association and it turned out they were looking for help with the accounts. That's my profession. My wife comes with me to the meetings, and she enjoys the company. We pop into the office two or three times a week and sometimes there are activities on that she can do while I'm toiling over the figures. A month ago we went to Parliament to a meeting to tell elected representatives about the needs of people with dementia. I feel a new lease of life. I didn't know about dementia before, but now I do I am determined to make the situation better for those coming after than they were for us. (John, retired accountant, 72)

In some languages there is not even a word for 'carer' because in that culture caring for someone when they are sick and vulnerable is simply what you do. We use the word in English because our system needs to identify the people who are doing the work of caring. There are 'carer's allowances' and 'carer's assessments' and 'carer support groups'. You can't access any of these unless you are identified as a carer. Organisations like Carers UK are there to help you with advice on caring … but also with companionship at what can be a lonely time. Their details are at the end of this book. In Scotland there is a website called Care Information (www.careinfoscotland.co.uk/home.aspx) and NHS Choices in England has a wealth of wide-ranging information for carers on their website (www.nhs.uk/CarersDirect/yourself/Pages/ Yourownwellbeinghome.aspx). This includes advice on getting time off work, types of carer breaks, how to take care of yourself, managing relationships and other issues, including hints for male carers who sometimes face practical problems because our society in general expects carers to be female, which is wrong. This advice is backed up by tools to assess your physical fitness and mental well-being. They take only moments to use and are connected to good advice about staying well. You have to look after yourself if you are going to be able to help others.

Chapter 4

Adjusting to the news: for people with dementia

I felt totally alone, with the world receding from me in every direction, and you could have used my anger to weld steel. (Terry Pratchett, October 2008, describing when he was diagnosed)

To say I understand what happens to someone when they are told they have dementia would be to trivialise a catastrophe that I have not yet experienced. It is not for me to say. When first diagnosed, my friends with dementia tell me, it's hard to find anything positive to say. Dementia is a bad thing. The Alzheimer Europe website gives reflections from people with dementia about how it was when they were diagnosed.

We were diagnosed over two years ago but can still remember those first shattering feelings – shock, disbelief, fear, shame, feeling cut off … and feeling very alone. Your brain feels numb and you can't take it all in … But take heart, these first terrible feelings really do pass. We know – we've been there. (Pat, James and Ian, www.alzheimer-europe. org/Living-with-dementia/After-diagnosis-What-next/Diagnosis-of-dementia/Facing-the-diagnosis)

The NHS Choices website says, 'Once the initial feelings of shock have passed, it is time to move on and create an action plan for the future.' In a breathtaking list of what you should do, it mentions such elements as making a will and putting your papers in order. It's the shock of the mundane. It does not say, 'We are so, so sorry.' But it should say that, because of what we know the health service might be about to do to you.

It is a strange life when you 'come out'. People get embarrassed, lower their voices, get lost for words ... It seems that when you have cancer you are a brave battler against the disease, but when you have Alzheimer's you are an old fart. That's how people see you. It makes you feel quite alone. (Terry Pratchett, discussing stigma in dementia)

People with dementia are often very angry, because in addition to the unfairness of the disease they are dismayed by the exclusion they experience, even when people are talking about dementia and about them.

It may be hard for people with dementia to speak out, but guidelines have been written with the help of people with dementia in order to offer guidance on this. The aim is to share good practice about the best ways of involving people with dementia. Dementia working groups have been set up, like The Forget Me Nots in Swindon. These people with dementia have been involved in making films about dementia. The SURF (Service User Reference Forum) group in Liverpool has worked on raising awareness in children and on innovative products that are being developed for people with dementia.

Alzheimer Europe brought together people with dementia to talk about what it means for them. Their words are in a manual entitled *Alzheimer's Disease: After the Diagnosis – What Next?* Dr James McKillop, MBE, who himself has a diagnosis of dementia, was instrumental in reviewing drafts of that manual (and this book) to make sure that the information is relevant and understandable. The message is clear. Dementia does not define people, though their powers will be limited in a range of ways over time. I am inspired by my friends with dementia who do what Winston Churchill advised at the end of every phone call during the Second World War: 'Keep buggering on.'

Sometimes angry people get organised and take collective action. An early group was the Scottish Dementia Working Group, a politically active forum made up of people with dementia. When undertaking a project called DEEP (the Dementia Engagement and Empowerment Project) in 2012,[*] the Joseph Rowntree Foundation discovered that there were not many groups led by or actively involving people with dementia that were influencing services and policies in England. That has changed radically and not only are there local groups, but there is guidance on how conferences and educational events should be organised to make sure that the voices of people with dementia are heard.

'Nothing about us without us' (EDUCATE Early Dementia Users Co-operative Aiming to Educate www.educatestockport.org.uk)

Being involved at the time when you are just coming to terms with a diagnosis can be difficult. Campaigning and activism are different from being in a support group, but those involved often say that the support from an action group and the sense of empowerment are really significant when other supports are fading away and power seems to have been stripped away from you. The friendship and camaraderie are important. Time, fatigue and cost have all been identified as barriers to involvement. At the Alzheimer Europe conference in Malta in 2013 a Czech woman with dementia, Nina Baláčková, spoke of her personal experience of dementia and what it was like being part of the European Working Group of People with Dementia. There

---

[*]See www.mentalhealth.org.uk/our-work/research/dementia-engagementand-empowerment-project for details.

was standing room only for her speech, and the place was filled with people with dementia, carers, care workers and researchers who were inspired and moved by the discussion. She said, 'You can't choose what you feel, but you can choose what you do with it.'

Other people with dementia are emphatic about the importance of living well.

While there are drawbacks, I still enjoy living. I meet so many interesting people I would never have met had I not had dementia. I bask in their genuine friendship. I do miss a regular wage and driving, but hey, people in graveyards would gladly change places with me. I savour the life I currently have. (James McKillop, founder member of the Scottish Dementia Working Group)

Anyone who wonders what it feels like to have dementia should look at the Alzheimer's Society forum for people who have dementia, where contributors talk to each other about how their day-to-day life is.

The emphasis in the public messages of the advocacy organisations is on living well with dementia. In recent years there has been a lot of concern about whether that message puts people under unnecessary pressure. It became difficult for people to say negative things about having dementia. Describing someone as 'suffering from dementia' became politically incorrect. In giving a voice and a stage to some untypical people diagnosed with dementia, the advocacy organisations have also exposed them to unwelcome questioning.

I mean, I don't want to be rude, but she's supposed to have dementia and she's been talking about it for fourteen years. I thought if it was a progressive disease she would have died by now. Do you think she's been wrongly diagnosed? She's certainly not typical, but she keeps turning up at conferences speaking on behalf of us all. But you don't like to say anything. The others get so angry. (Person with dementia speaking about another)

So even in dementia diagnosis there are politics and argument, but the most important message is that there is life. Whether you want to keep it private or get on the road to campaign, there are still choices that you can make for yourself. In aircraft safety announcements you are told to put on your own oxygen mask before assisting other people. On ferries you are told to put on your own life jacket first. Remember to take care of yourself, otherwise you won't be able to help support others or participate in raising awareness and getting real political action on dementia. Tell other people that they must help you, and if they don't know how, recommend some of the later chapters in this book.

Chapter 5

What are friends for?

A friend is someone who knows the song in your heart and can sing it back to you when you have forgotten the words.

Dementia presents a particular problem to friends if you are not part of the family. You might not know much about it yourself and the whole idea of it is terrifying. You want to help, but you are afraid of being embarrassing or inappropriate and you just don't know what would make a difference. Reading this chapter will provide guidance on what often does make a difference, based on what people with dementia and their family carers say.

We often get advised to 'keep up with friends'. This is the first time I've seen advice for friends to help. It is so badly needed, why has it not been done before? The Government and local authorities will have to take notice as it can save them a lot of care costs. (James McKillop)

Simple and easy-to-implement ideas for helping and staying with a friend through this dark time are presented here, together with scenarios that are a bit tricky, and also illustrations of how to cope and hints for how to have a conversation and be with people who have dementia.

Treat us as normal people. We're still here, just a little slower and sometimes confused.

This quote is from the Alzheimer's Disease International *World Alzheimer's Report* 2012,* which focused on the times and the places where awkwardness, humiliation and shame are associated with dementia. The report brought to light some important views from carers of people with dementia who if they were writing this would say:

- I do want and need help.
- I spend more time on caring than you think.
- I am isolated by my twenty-four-hour responsibility.
- I am judged by the rest of my family for the quality of my caring.
- I may not take the initiative in keeping up with our relationship.
- I may not be able to afford some of the support that is available.
- I have health and stress problems because I am a carer.

If people with dementia who were interviewed for the report were writing this they would say:

- I am aware that you are afraid to talk to me.
- I would like to be included in conversations.
- I would encourage you to ask me about whether I want to discuss memory loss, because I might often want to.
- I know my own limitations.
- I want you to ask me if I want you to help me remember words I forget.
- I would often prefer you not to correct what I say, but show me you understand the meaning.
- I am disheartened when you avoid or ignore me.

---

* See www.alz.co.uk/research/WorldAlzheimerReport2012.pdf.

- I am humiliated when you talk to my relative and not to me.
- I don't want to be a burden, so I hold myself back from things I'd like to do with you.
- I won't be taking the initiative as much any more.

As a friend who wants to help, you can do no better than respond to what the carers and people with dementia say.

What the carers would say

I do want and need help

If you want to help, it's really important to ask what would be most helpful. It might not be what you imagine. You might think getting in a bit of shopping would be good, when in fact shopping is the one outing the carer has to look forward to. Maybe they'd rather have a lift to the shops, or they'd rather that you stay in the house with the person with dementia while they go out shopping on their own.

You will see in Chapter 8 that one of the most important things for staying well for a person with dementia is exercise. Just think, if you offer to take them for a walk when you are taking your dog out (or push them in a wheelchair if they are beyond walking), you can get four times the benefit. Dog enjoys walk, person with dementia gets health benefits, carer gets an hour of respite and you get exercise! What's not to love about that? You might even help them sleep that night, which makes five benefits. It is the gift that keeps giving.

Doing activities with the person with dementia supports the carer with their burden. 'Burden' is such an awful word, because it sounds like something you'd want to put down. The carer does not always want to put it down.

I'm not her carer. She's my wife. After fifty-five years I could not sleep without her in the bed beside me. Why would I want her to be in a home? (Frederick, 79)

There is no end to the list of useful chores you can do, including help with the garden, doing care and repair jobs, help with forms and correspondence, transport to church, taking round a batch of pancakes or a pot roast once a week, pulling out the bin for the collection, lending the latest DVD movie – being a friend in need. Not being sexist, but there are plenty of 'man' jobs and 'woman' jobs and you can make up for the gender imbalance in their house. If the man with dementia used to deal with the hedge cutting, be a hero and do it for him.

I spend more time on caring than you think

The best of our good friends have no idea how much time this takes up. If the carer goes out to work, they may spend hours there worrying, or making phone calls, or altering their work pattern to fit in with caring. Even if they have retired or had to give up their job, the carer may be woken up many times in the night and so is still exhausted. If you as a friend can give this person the gift of time, you will be doing the best you can. Time is rationed, and the carer does not have enough to guarantee their mental and physical health and personal safety. Donate time. You can do this either by house-sitting during the day, to let them get out, or at night, to let them sleep. You can undertake time-consuming tasks for them, using up some of your own free time. You can take the person with dementia away for long enough to give the carer a break. Encourage them to use the time for something that will really recharge their batteries. A play, a movie, a concert … these are nice highbrow activities. But to be honest some carers can't even use the toilet without being interrupted, so don't be surprised if they seem not to have done what you'd think of as 'much' with the time. A shower, a shave and an uninterrupted visit to the loo might be a real treat for a gentleman whose wife clings to him like a limpet, even following him into the toilet.

I am isolated by my twenty-four-hour responsibility

Sometimes just being there and listening to the carer is helpful. If you take round that batch of pancakes, demand a cup of tea and eat some together. You don't even have to go over if there is no time or your friend lives far away. There are excellent international examples of low-level support for isolated carers in the form of a regular phone call. Every morning the person gets a call from someone asking the usual things. How was your night? Are you doing anything today? How are you both? Did you see *Strictly Come Dancing* last night? Has this politician no shame? Why is the weather not as good as it was when we were young? Not many of us can survive for days without speaking to anyone other than the stranger who is emerging in our own home as dementia takes hold. A regular phone call can be a lifeline.

It may be that the carer already has Skype and is familiar with electronic forms of communication, but if not you can help set them up. Of course they are not as good as being in the room with someone, but they open a window that people at the other side can use, like friends and family from far away. That window might be closed if you don't help the person to get online.

When you are inviting a carer to come out with you, or come to your house, make sure that they understand the person with dementia is welcome as well, and take care of both. I know that group meetings of carers might sound grim to you, if the people have nothing at all in common other than caring, but it can be incredibly useful. Help your friend to find and attend such a group if they want to.

I knew Alison had vascular dementia but it was only when someone said, 'Ask the Alzheimer's Society,' that I realised they've got a meeting I can go to. I met a man just like me and his wife was the same as Alison. He did make me laugh. He says I made him feel better because he felt less alone. Now his wife has passed away he comes round sometimes and entices me out to the pub – not that I need much persuasion. (Frederick, 79)

I am judged by the rest of my family for the quality of my caring

I've been going in to see Mum every day for two years, making her tea every night on the way home from work, before going home to cook for the kids and my man. Recently she got even more frail and it was taking longer and longer. I eventually had to get social services to get carers in to do the morning and evening for me on weekdays, and I go and do a big clear-up at the weekend and bathe and feed her then. Then I got this horrible phone call from my sister because she had called in and found strangers in the house. It's the first time she's visited in six months but she was horrible to me, calling me names and blaming me. (S.M., daughter)

The tension in families can be appalling, and if you are a friend you may have to listen to quite a lot of this. Hindsight is a wonderful thing and it might not help your relationship if you point out that it would have been a good idea to let the sister know about the change of circumstances. At least you now know the lie of the land, that the sister is unhelpfully oversensitive in one way and unhelpfully insensitive in another way, and if your friend is making any other changes you can prompt her to let the rest of the family know, galling though such a responsibility might seem to her.

I not only have to do it all, but I have to report back to the lazy cow as well! (S.M.)

Families can start a private blog or WhatsApp group where everyone has their own responsibility to log in and find out for themselves what is going on. Keeping a diary of what is happening on top of everything else might seem a burden, but it has a number of benefits, including reminding everyone how much change has taken place.

Families accuse each other of terrible crimes, and think that the carer is 'doing them out of' inheritance, or affection or things we can't even imagine. Of course if you thought the carer was abusing the person with dementia you'd inform the authorities. If you are not sure how to go about this you can contact Action on Elder Abuse which has a website and a helpline. But if they are not and you are their friend, listen, listen and then listen some more. And find a way of sympathising without throwing fuel on the fire. Two years from now the mother may be dead and those sisters will need to be the best support they can be for each other.

I may not take the initiative in keeping up with our relationship

If you invite someone a few times and they never take you up on the offer, the usual response is to take the hint and drop them. Once they have missed sending you a birthday or Christmas card a few times, you start to erase their name from your own list. You might just realise one day that you've not spoken for a year or two. Always, always be the one who makes the contact, if they are struggling with dementia in their family. The amount of time that they have is severely limited. Being with you might be a treat that they have denied themselves. The exhaustion from their tasks may give them the idea that they don't have time to wash and dress well enough to come out with you for a coffee, even if they could leave their loved one at home alone. Shame about the state their house is in might stop them, out of pride, from inviting you round.

If you are a friend you will know ways around this problem. Be patient and persistent and remember that this is not about you. Carers tell us that friends just stop calling and they are embarrassed to beg for attention. Socialising is one of the few activities that make a difference in dementia, so do it for the person with dementia if not for the carer. You can help both at once.

I may not be able to afford some of the support that is available

Reading Chapter 10 might be a revelation when you realise that, in spite of our internationally once envied health and social care system in the UK, there are many services that would be useful that have to be paid for, even if they come through the local council. If you are wondering why the person does not take up everything that is available, consider whether finance may be an issue.

Our house is worth a lot of money, I know, but there's not much cash now our investments are getting no returns. If I sell the house, she'll be even more confused by the move. We look rich but I can't afford the home help. I'm not having that means test. (Pat, 85, sister of Helen, 81)

Many older people avoid social services and social work departments because they are afraid that they'll lose control of the situation. As a friend you could do them a favour by making sure that they know about the 'wealth check' that can be done discreetly and privately by a charity like Age UK, through which they can find ways of maximising their income they did not previously know about. A huge number of allowances are never collected by carers. A family lawyer could help here, if they could afford the fee. But a social work assessment is a legal right, and that can help uncover possible affordable sources of help.

In addition, think of free or low-cost things that you can do together. If you invite them out for a meal they might say no because they can't pay or return the compliment if you pay. On the other hand, you could go for a walk in the park together, or attend the local farmer's market or shopping centre just to window shop, or go to church ... or any other free stuff.

I have health and stress problems because I am a carer

The research on stress and burden is extensive, but different people have different coping skills, so their profound commitment is not necessarily going to make them ill. Of the people who do get ill, they seem to have more health problems as the person with dementia gets more dementia problems. Many carer health problems can be reversed if they are given proper information and support. Just by being a good friend you can reduce the risk of this person having health and stress problems. You can help gather information and find out where there are other sources of support. And of course you can just be there for them.

Carers are a diverse bunch of people. They're not recruited against a job description and skills set. The timescale of their caring is relevant. In the run-up to getting a diagnosis there has been a worrying time for them and it can be a relief to know what was causing the problems. Conversely, the time when the person goes into a care home, which some might think of as a relief, is a time of terrible loss and change, and constant worry about whether the home is doing the care right. Friends can help with the transition, and then you could take turns at visiting the home, or use the new-found free time to be a friend again in the old ways, going out and about. Remember that even when they are in a home, the person with dementia can still be entertained by you, on or off the premises.

What the people with dementia would say

I am aware that you are afraid to talk to me

To be honest, they've got more to be afraid of than you do. Imagine how it feels when someone vaguely familiar is coming towards you and you are searching for their name. It happens to all of us – at work, at a party, in the street. Your main concern is whether you are going to embarrass yourself.

You may be afraid of getting something wrong, but the person with dementia is at a stage in their life when they are getting lots and lots of things wrong, and remembering your face might just be another one of them. So save them from that. Walk up and introduce yourself. If you are really clever you can do it in a way that does not draw attention to the problem.

Doris and I were standing at the post office together and Ethel, who has dementia, came in. I said to Ethel when she got close to us, 'Hello, Ethel, how are you? Look, Doris, here is Ethel.' And Doris replied, 'How are you today? John and I were nearly late for church on Sunday.' I followed up by saying, 'Well, Ethel. You can tell everyone at the church that Doris and John are going to try to be on time.' We all laughed, and Ethel was nudged to remember that we are John and Doris she knows from the church. We don't usually use our own names much in conversation, but we make a point with Ethel, and we plant clues in what we say. If everyone did that she'd be able to join in more often. (Doris and John, friends of Ethel, 61)

As a busy professor in the dementia field, I meet thousands of people every year and I occasionally don't remember someone from a few months ago, or whom I met only briefly. The person I meet often assumes that I'll remember them better than I do, and it's embarrassing, because I don't want to insult anyone. That's a hazard of my job, and I find ways round it. However, a friend of someone with dementia would do their best to reduce the problems for them, so keep introducing yourself even when it seems a bit silly. Err on the right side.

I would like to be included in conversations

I remember how you made me feel …

To begin with there will not be a lot of change from what you are used to in your friend, but by the end the person may not have much language left. Dementia spreads over a number of years, so the way of speaking with a person with dementia will change over time.

I myself find that I need things repeated as I did not hear them properly. I might have misheard a word which throws the whole sentence out. I usually turn to Maureen, who repeats the question and I can follow her voice. I am used to it. With some individuals I never know what they said and we always have to get Maureen to repeat for me. (James McKillop)

As the words disappear, non-verbal communication becomes more and more important. A hug, a handshake, linked arms or hands – all of these can communicate something right to the end. Smiles and just sitting together can be a great comfort.

However, if you want to converse remember the following:

- The language difficulties will vary according to the type of dementia, but in general over time you need to leave more time for questions and comments to sink in, and for responses to come back. Relax – it's the quality that counts, not the speed! (A great revelation for me was listening to a tape of a friend with dementia talking. When I played it at twice normal speed, he sounded coherent and fluent. When I had listened at normal speed, I wondered if he was making sense. My impatience with his speed of communication was making me judgemental about the content of what he was saying.)

- A person with frontotemporal dementia may start to say things that are a bit shocking or to use language that could be offensive. A friend will respond to what is good in what someone says, so don't respond to what you think of as bad. There is no point in starting an argument about whether they should curse. It's the illness talking.

- Although it is important to keep your conversation at the right pace, and that is probably slower than your normal pace, avoid the risk of sounding like a primary school teacher talking to a child. It's not appreciated and it doesn't help. A friend must not treat you like a wally, even if you have dementia.

- A person with dementia does not lose their sense of humour. My friends with dementia are among the funniest people I've been with. They flirt and tell rude jokes and are politically incorrect as much as the next person. Don't try to sanctify them.

- Here is a controversial point. I always say that if a person with dementia has not understood something, it's a good idea to say the same thing again. The Alzheimer's Society says rephrase it. Maybe they are assuming that the friend said the first thing in a way that is too complicated and so needs to simplify it.

Sometimes you do just need to say it again, and if you say it again differently, the person then wonders what they missed when you first spoke. You know the person, so just try what works.

● Listen very carefully and take time. I've found that even if the person sounds incoherent at first, when you stick with it the meaning does come out. It is like they are talking in 'Scribble'.

My grandmother used to behave as if she was chattering away, with mixed-up words, exclamations, nods and winks, and then a clear phrase would come through, out of context, like a clearing in fog that opened and closed again just as quick. We used to say she was talking in 'Scribble', a new sort of jumbled-up language which had real meaning to her. (J.M., granddaughter)

● Crowded places are difficult for chatting. Background noise makes attention really difficult in dementia, so don't try to have a big conversation in a crowded or busy place, and even in a domestic setting switch off the radio or TV in order to talk properly.

I would encourage you to ask me about whether I want to discuss memory loss, because I might often want to

As a friend of a person with dementia, you may well have read a bit about it. You are clearly reading this book anyway. So you probably want to know what kind of dementia it is, and what is likely to happen next. You might be afraid to ask because the answer might be distressing. We also have a natural reserve about personal questions. People are always talking about their own illnesses and their friends' illnesses, and keep gall stones in a jar on the mantelpiece, but there is something intimate and potentially shameful about a 'mental' condition. If you are a friend you might be one of the few people that I can share my hopes and fears with. It might be that I want to talk to you about stuff I can't share with my family. At least let me know that you have an open door for that sort of conversation. And respect it if I say that my door is firmly closed. Things might change over time, though.

I know my own limitations

People sometimes wonder if the person with dementia is unaware of what is happening to them. More and more evidence is appearing that demonstrates they do know, and for much longer than we might think. In fact some people know that something is going wrong long before they can persuade a doctor or anyone else that they've got this problem. When you see the lengths to which people will go to conceal the impairments that are hitting them, it's clear that they know. The earlier the diagnosis, the more chance they have of finding out about the condition, what can be done to keep symptoms at bay and what the prognosis is.

The day after I got my diagnosis everybody started treating me like an idiot. (Arlene, 73)

As a friend, of course you will be worried about whether they'll get lost, or be swindled by people in shops, or let strangers into the house to rob them. But the person with dementia should be your guide as to what they can do. People with dementia are entitled to take risks and make unwise decisions – it's not up to their friends, and a good friend can support them in doing what they really want. You might have to help them stand up to others.

I want you to ask me if I want you to help me remember words I forget

The advice that is given when you are talking to a friend with dementia is not unlike the advice for talking to someone who has another communication disorder, stuttering. Relax and take time. Don't raise your voice, because the problem is not deafness. Use normal eye contact: a hard stare would be really disconcerting, and you need to realise that your facial expression will be read and recognised by your friend, so be aware of it. Listen and show that you are listening with genuine interest and are not making judgements. If you interrupt and don't let them finish their turn at speaking it will be demoralising. One problem in dementia is difficulty in finding words, and some people think it is really helpful if you offer the word. Others find it depressing, because they believe that straining to find the word will make them better at finding other words – like a memory-strengthening exercise. If you 'find' the wrong word persistently you are going to be really annoying, so ask them what is most helpful and do what they want.

I would often prefer you not to correct what I say, but show me you understand the meaning

My gran used to talk to me in 'Scribble'. The words were all mixed up or made up. But if you looked in her eyes and listened to her tone you could tell what she was saying. 'Thank you for these beautiful flowers' … or 'Where's Grandad, I really miss him' … or 'I wonder who you are, but I think you're a kind girl' … We could be together for hours like that. It reminded me of the 'concrete poems' they used to teach us at school in the Sixties. The intended effect of those was never in the literal meaning of the actual words used. (J.M., granddaughter)

Depending on the cause of the dementia, the words used by a person may start to seem unintelligible. When professionals sometimes say, 'She can't communicate,' they really mean, 'She can't communicate verbally in a way that I understand.' Verbal communication is not all it is cracked up to be. Ask any cat – they do fine without it. Remember that the person with dementia is even more dependent on non-verbal communication and still can read it, even if you can't. A sigh of exasperation or rolling of the eyes, which are unconscious movements on your part, will communicate themselves very clearly to the apparently uncommunicative person before you. They'll read you like a book. Try to respond to your friend's version of 'Scribble'. Or get them a cat.

When your friend with dementia says no one ever comes to visit her, don't argue the fact that carers come in three times a day, and the vicar once a week, and the daughter every evening and you are standing there, living proof of visitors. Listen to the meaning underneath the words. What she is saying is that she feels abandoned and it does not matter at that moment that she's really not been abandoned. Work with what she feels and do something to distract her from that feeling for at least the time you are together. Talk about the past, show pictures, sing a song, walk round the garden … just be together. Pray or meditate if that is what you would always have done. People with dementia get a really interesting emotional hangover in that, if you upset them, they remain upset after they've forgotten what upset them. If you comfort and distract them happily, they remain happy long after they've forgotten your kindness and humour. You can help them to be happy even after you have gone.

I am disheartened when you avoid or ignore me

A friend would not stay away from a person with dementia. It is really helpful if you pay attention and offer companionship and kindness. Although this section is intended to be positive and practical, I know it is a tough gig being cheerful and friendly for someone who is losing their cognitive capacity and who might at some stage not even remember who you are. But you've got many options. If it is too hard to be with them for long and try to communicate, you can do something for their carers. People go out and support charities and walk the Great Wall of China to raise money in memory of people with dementia who were their friends. Somewhere, somehow, they will know that you are doing this and be grateful. Anyone can do that, but only a friend can take you for a round of golf, and not worry about the fact that you can't keep the score any more and sometimes face the wrong direction. A visit can make a difference, even though you might not think so at the time.

When I was in the Guides we had to do the 'visitor' badge test. It involved picking a solitary person we knew and going round to see them. I picked a retired schoolteacher who had taught me in primary school. I was about sixteen. Looking back, I can see that she had dementia. She never knew I was coming even though it was all arranged. She would offer me tea and then not make it. She repeated the same things she'd said before. She'd even go out of the room and leave me alone and forget that I was in her house. Now I realise that what seemed like a futile box-ticking exercise for my badge was probably a really good thing. She was hard to visit, and as a result everyone else in her circle was ignoring her. I went six times and I wish now I'd kept it up. (Dementia nurse)

I am humiliated when you talk to my relative and not to me

The 'Does he take sugar?' cliché has entered our language as an expression for the syndrome where able-bodied people are unable to speak directly to a person with a disability. Friends may be embarrassed and even ashamed to catch the eye of the person with dementia. It is as if there might be something showing in their face, like pity or horror, which they don't want the person with dementia to see. You just have to get over that. Spend time if you need it talking about your horror with someone else, and prepare yourself to be with your friend without showing dismay. After all, this is their tragedy, not yours, and for once this is a tragedy with which you can help.

The person with dementia is often stripped of their dignity, even at the early stages of the condition, so you can be a role model for everyone else about how they should be supported and regarded properly. There is even a tendency for family themselves to start speaking for the person with dementia before this is remotely necessary. You can help with this by your example.

When someone with dementia makes jokes about dementia itself, the power base shifts. The potential for humiliation is reversed and people who are sanctimonious about dementia are put in their place. Fiona Phillips in the *Mirror* newspaper talked about Tony Booth, an actor who had dementia, and his contribution to a dementia meeting.

*He walks in, a huge smile on his still-handsome face, accompanied by former teacher Stephanie, his fourth wife. His addictions now reduced to cigarettes and tea, he raises his cuppa and cheekily proclaims, 'I'll drink to that,' as the aims of the session are outlined. When the Alzheimer's Society volunteer asks the group, 'What do you think of when you see the word dementia?', always looking for a laugh, he shouts out, 'I've forgotten!' Later his eyes twinkle as he asks, 'Is it true that men drive women demented?' Much hilarity ensues ... (*Mirror, 10 February 2014)

His ebullient personality was intact, so no one was going to talk to his wife about him in his presence. You need to be sure you don't do this accidentally to a less confident personality.

I don't want to be a burden, so I hold myself back from things I'd like to do with you

You may need to use strong encouragement to get the person to join in, because they have a fear of holding everyone back. They might want to join you on a trip abroad but be afraid to ask. They might want to climb one last mountain but feel that the responsibility for them is something you can't take on. They won't come to the club with you any more in case they embarrass themselves and you. As a friend you may influence the person with abundant demonstrations of attention and friendliness. Their self-esteem is low and their self-confidence even lower, so you will have to work hard to help them understand they are not a burden. The confidence of their friends will help make up for their own lack of confidence.

The strongest expression of this urge to avoid being a burden would be the inclination to attempt suicide. In the Netherlands dementia can be a justification for euthanasia, which is sad because the law requires you to die before you are overtaken by the dementia, and while you are relatively well. And by the later stages of dementia, there is no diminution in the human instinct to stay alive. In July 2018 a doctor there was reprimanded for persuading a family to hold down a woman with dementia who was resisting euthanasia, having once asked for it. There is evidence that people with nightmare conditions such as motor neurone disease, faced with the horror of not being able to breathe or swallow, might consider suicide, or people with uncontrolled pain feel that they personally cannot bear to live with it. However, there is no evidence that people with dementia are actually more suicidal than other older people. But there are those who have thought they ought to be.

Elderly people suffering from dementia should consider ending their lives because they are a burden on the NHS and their families, according to the influential medical ethics expert Baroness Warnock. The veteran Government adviser said pensioners in mental decline are 'wasting people's lives' because of the care they require and should be allowed to opt for euthanasia even if they are not in pain ... Lady Warnock ... [is] a former headmistress who went on to become Britain's leading moral philosopher ... (Daily Telegraph, *18 September 2008*)

I can think of nothing more tragic than where someone wants to kill themselves because of the burden they are to other people. Other people have given them the view that they are a burden and friends can lessen that. So do everything you can to show that your friend with dementia is not a burden and have fun doing the things you both like.

The idea is to die young as late as possible (Ashley Montagu, anthropologist)

I won't be taking the initiative as much any more

The final point is that you need to keep going even when you've reached the position where you are not sure that they know you. We do this out of humanity and self-respect, as much as for the benefit of our friends. This is what being human is. Being a friend right up till the end of life is the most precious gift in the world.

I felt privileged to be allowed to be involved and to help in looking after her a bit and supporting her husband. He's such a lovely man and he cared for her so beautifully. He deserved all the help and respect I could give him. (John, friend)

There are many practical tasks you can do to help, like undertaking simple chores, picking up prescriptions or fetching a newspaper. If you are the carer, don't hesitate to ask friends to help. But just being there is really important.

Piglet sidled up to Pooh from behind.

'Pooh?' he whispered.

'Yes, Piglet?'

'Nothing,' said Piglet, taking Pooh's hand. 'I just wanted to be sure of you.'

(A. A. Milne)

Chapter 6

How to keep dementia at bay

There are problems in providing evidence for some of the claims that are made about how to delay dementia. The reporting of research sometimes gives rise to conflicting results. It is really challenging to design a research programme, for example, that tests the effect of only vitamins and not exercise, or only fish and not stress. As a result, studies appear to contradict each other, because the researchers were not measuring the same things, and they were not able to narrow their focus enough. Doing research on humans is complicated because we are complicated. Before listing what is said to help, it is worth noting that this is your excuse to focus on the elements here that you like best and can stick with. Take your pick, because most of it probably helps a bit. If you are interested in prevention and staying well, the thing for which there is the strongest evidence is exercise. That is one of the important messages in this chapter, but everything else described here will make some difference to nearly everyone.

Since the first edition of this book, a new set of guidelines has been produced by the World Health Organization on risk reduction. They are summarised in the epilogue at the end of this book. The emphasis is on what systems should be doing to help people and it is described as a 'tool for healthcare providers as well as governments', but it will be useful for individuals to act

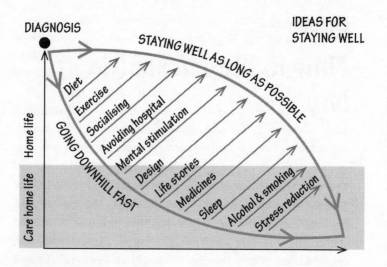

independently or to ask your health provider for things that will help you to reduce the risk of decline in your brain.

The disease vs. the symptoms

The information available on the internet and in newspapers is sometimes confusing, because the journalist or reporter does not explain or perhaps even understand that there is a difference between 'Alzheimer's disease' (or Pick's disease, or vascular, or any other disease process – see Chapter 1) and 'symptoms of dementia'. So when they highlight a new wonder food or activity that can 'slow Alzheimer's disease' they might be talking about slowing the rate of build-up of the plaques and tangles in the anatomy of the brain, or they might specifically be talking about slowing up the dementia symptoms. It is hard to follow the news when journalists use 'Alzheimer's' as a synonym for any 'dementia', no matter what the cause, and when they don't distinguish between the different symptoms, like memory loss, difficulty in working things out, stress reactions, difficulty in learning new things, etc. And sometimes the experiment turns out to have been on mice only so far, which is encouraging. But it is frankly misleading if the headline implies that it's about humans.

The most definitive clinical measure of the underlying *disease* process unfortunately comes only from weighing and dissecting the brain tissue at post-mortem. Because dementia *symptoms* are about worrying changes in how a person is behaving and thinking, you can see whether those symptoms have increased or decreased while the person is still alive. The measuring of 'dementia symptoms' is done by clinicians and researchers using a wide range of tests. They choose which of the individual dementia symptoms, or which groups of symptoms, are most relevant to their study and use a test that measures those specific symptoms. The report in the newspaper may say that an intervention 'reduces Alzheimer's' when the research actually demonstrates only that it improves one particular symptom of dementia, such as memory. You can help with memory problems, one symptom of dementia, without reducing the Alzheimer's disease. And you can reduce one symptom of dementia, without affecting other symptoms of dementia. The memory might be better, but the aggression and agitation might not have improved at all. Pharmaceutical researchers are particularly interested in memory, but it might be that an intervention that fails to improve memory makes something else (that is harder to measure) better.

This patient was tested to see if the medication was making any difference to her and the standard cognition tests were negative. Not enough improvement to make it worth the cost of the prescription. Then the family pointed out that since she got the medication she had started to play the piano again, having stopped doing that for a long time. From the research measurement point of view the medication was not working; but it transformed her in a way that mattered to her, and to the family. So can we say it did not work? (Abridged from a clinical report by Professor Kenneth Rockwood, Dalhousie University, Canada)

From a practical point of view we have to ask which makes a difference to the patient – slowing the underlying disease or slowing the symptoms? Personally, I do not care if my brain shrinks a bit as long as it is not too noticeable in my daily life. It's of no benefit to me if the medication stops the brain shrinking but my mental capacity continues to shrink. What matters to me is the quality of my daily life.

There are some interventions that may affect the underlying diseases and there are some interventions that affect only the symptoms. For example, later in this book you will find advice on increasing light levels in the place where you live. That does not affect the rate at which the brain shrinks, but it does reduce the amount of dementia symptoms experienced by the person. It would be good to try to do both, but while the scientists are struggling with the former, you can still roll up your sleeves and get on with the latter. There is something practical that you can do.

The things that you can do that we think keep dementia at bay are worth sticking with (or starting) even if you already have a diagnosis. They will help you to stay well, and so keeping them up as long as possible is a really good idea.

Drugs

I will do anything in my power to help them find a medicine for dementia, even if it is too late for me. (Volunteer with dementia in the Scottish Dementia Clinical Network cohort)

- There is no medicine that will prevent the development of the underlying diseases that cause dementia, except those medicines that will help with conditions like depression, high blood pressure, raised cholesterol, diabetes, etc. If you have any of those conditions your treatment for them and management of them are important, because all of them predispose a person to developing dementia.

- Pharmaceutical companies have been looking very hard for a drug or vaccine to prevent dementia, because the financial rewards of such a discovery would be amazing, apart from the humanitarian issues. This is why you might get cross when people complain that they have found a homely 'cure' like coconut oil and no one is listening to them. Believe me, if there was anything in it, they'd be better keeping quiet until they get the patents sorted out. We all want it and it's worth a fortune.

- Many of the drug trials for Alzheimer's disease have been discontinued by big pharmaceutical companies. The chance of success is so slim they've judged that it is not worth their time to continue.

- The medication that is currently licensed for use in the UK for dementia (acetylcholinesterase inhibitors) is mainly for the Alzheimer's form of dementia and is usually prescribed in the early and middle stages of the disease, when the maximum benefit is derived from them. This is a primary reason why early diagnosis is seen to be a good idea by doctors and this has helped to get an increase in access to diagnosis. The aim of the medication is to stabilise the condition. Not everybody will benefit from these drugs. They have side effects, including nausea and vomiting, and they can lower the pulse rate. Memantine hydrochloride is used to treat severe Alzheimer's disease or sometimes for moderate cases that don't respond to acetylcholinesterase inhibitors. It is often said that they only delay the progress of symptoms, but they also appear to have an impact on the pathology that underlies the diseases that cause the symptoms. Cynical people say that the campaign to get people diagnosed early is purely to do with increasing drug company profits, but I don't agree.

Smoking and alcohol

The gentlemen who live here now have had difficult lives. Their families and former friends, often because of behaviours in the past that were a result of use of alcohol, reject them. We do not ask questions or judge them. Some of them cannot remember what happened three minutes ago but will tell you in great detail about a drinking party they had on their eighteenth birthday. The degradation of their faculties and what they have lost is tragic. Their limited lives are in sharp contrast with the macho culture which gave rise to their disabilities ... [In response to a question] Yes, many of them have military backgrounds and had distinguished service careers in theatres of war. (Matron of care home)

- Don't smoke. It would be better if you never had, but improvements will start the day you give up. There is clear evidence of this in the case of heavy smokers. If you give up in middle age, the risk of dementia after twenty years is the same as if you had never smoked. There is an obvious link with vascular health, but smoking is linked to risk of Alzheimer's disease as well.

- Alcohol-related brain damage (ARBD) is a preventable form of dementia. Women's brains are more vulnerable to alcohol and women who drink 'in moderation' have an increased risk of mild cognitive impairment. People who indulge in binge drinking, such as having a heavy session once a month, are more likely to experience problems. Fortnightly bingeing doubles the risk. People of all ages need to take care, but drinking in older age presents its own problems. There is research that has claimed to show that having one glass of red wine a day can have beneficial effects. I prefer champagne. Fortunately, recent research from the University of Reading suggests that people over forty would be wise to drink two or three glasses of bubbly a week. Hurrah! That research was done with rats, but I don't care. It's good enough evidence for me.

● If the management of drinking and smoking is challenging for you, remember that there are helplines and organisations there to support you that you can contact via your GP or searching the internet for your local support group.

There is a real problem with understanding research results. Often even the researcher doesn't recognise the reports in the media as their own research. By the time it has been through the press office of the University and passed to the sub-editor of the website, it is entirely changed. People are inclined to believe what suits them, and papers are inclined to report anything as 'surprising'. So a lot of it is nonsense. (Dementia academic)

Previous education

● The potential role of previous education is really interesting. If you examine brains after people have died, you can see 'neurodegeneration' (death of cell structures) and vascular damage, whether or not the person had dementia symptoms while alive. The amount of damage might be the same, no matter how much previous education the person had. The fascinating finding is that if the person did have a lot of formal education they could have had quite a lot of cell death and vascular damage while still not demonstrating dementia symptoms. So studying and becoming highly educated do not stop you getting Alzheimer's disease or vascular disease, but they will help you to cope with that damage happening inside your skull if it does. Mrs Thatcher with her two degrees and her busy mental life did get dementia, but arguably she would have been much worse much sooner if she'd left school at age eleven. Her highly developed and well-used brain was able to compensate for the damage.

More education did not protect individuals from developing neurodegenerative and vascular neuropathology by the time they died but it did appear to mitigate the impact of pathology on the clinical expression of dementia before death. The findings suggest that an understanding of the mechanisms leading to functional protection in the presence of pathology may be of considerable value to society. (Professor Carol Brayne)*

Speaking more than one language seems to offer some protection. There is some benefit in learning, even later in life. It's not about using a vocabulary app on your phone and practising alone. It seems to be related to the social aspect of learning more than one culture and different ways of expressing ideas.

Exercise

● It is well known that exercise reduces stress, boosts your mood and increases energy, but you may not realise that it actually appears to increase the physical amount of grey matter in your brain. The evidence for this in the research literature is very strong, much stronger than the evidence for some of the other suggested interventions here. If you take exercise, even

---

* See C. Brayne et al., 'Education, the Brain and Dementia: Neuroprotection or Compensation?', *Brain*, 133 (2010), pp. 2210–16.

in middle age, it reduces the dementia risk and improves your scores if you have MCI. It protects your brain and slows the decline and reduces the risk of those mini-strokes that cause vascular dementia.

- When thinking of a sport to take part in, avoid boxing or anything that involves repeatedly banging your head, like heading a heavy football. Older adults who have had even relatively mild brain injury have an increased risk of dementia. There is no evidence that a single mild injury increases the risk, but the more severe it is and the more repeated, the greater the risk. It might even be that some people have a genetic predisposition to this connection between a bang on the head and dementia. Wear your helmet when cycling. And we think a head blow in boxing should incur a foul penalty if we can't ban boxing altogether.

- Balance and coordination exercises are useful for all older people if you want to avoid the experience of falling and perhaps sustaining a fracture that will get you admitted to hospital. People with MCI may have balance and coordination problems more than the general population. Yoga and t'ai chi seem to work well for improving these functions. In vascular dementia problems with walking or balancing can occur at an earlier stage than in Alzheimer's. Starting from a higher level of fitness will help you to cope with any deterioration.

- Exercise does not need to be solitary or violent. Half an hour five days a week could make a difference. It needs only be of moderate intensity. The exercise you are most likely to keep up is the exercise that you enjoy. Socialising is really important also, so if you can combine the two that's great. Think of dancing. You socialise, you take exercise and with a bit of luck you get a glass of wine. Gardening is also good for you.

- Oxygen is the fuel for your brain and if your blood supply is compromised at all, then it is well worth doing anything you can to improve the circulation of your blood and its quality. If you make your heart and blood system more efficient, it will make your brain more efficient. Also consider the air quality in your house or where you live. Stuffy is bad.

- Exercise is magic for avoiding most health problems. Not managing those problems, for example high blood pressure, makes it more likely that you'll get dementia. There is even a link between obesity and dementia, so get moving in any way that you can, as the exercise will help with weight loss. As many as half of the cases of vascular dementia occur in people with high blood pressure, and exercise reduces your blood pressure. Small studies have indicated that taking blood pressure tablets reduces the risk of dementia, even in Alzheimer's disease.

One woman who corresponded with me was scathing about our support of exercise as a preventive, describing how poorly her husband is with dementia, and he was a professional athlete. It was important to explain that exercise is only one element of prevention. But later she revealed that he had been a footballer, and the combination of 'heading' a heavy wet leather ball and a history of subsequent alcohol use told a different story. (Dementia nurse)

Diet

- A 'Mediterranean' diet is one that is rich in nuts, fish and vegetables. It should contain plenty of fresh produce and less high-fat dairy and red meat than we have been accustomed to take. In studies, people who ate the Mediterranean way were less likely to develop dementia, but it is not clear what the connection is. There is no one lifestyle change or dietary change that will eliminate the risk. We need to eat good food in addition to the other interventions to stay well.

- Fibre is famous for reducing constipation and constipation can make you confused, particularly if you are already vulnerable to confusion because you've got some Alzheimer's or vascular damage. It is only in food that comes from plants. There are two types, soluble and insoluble. Soluble fibre can be digested by your body and helps to reduce the amount of cholesterol in your bloodstream. Your body makes cholesterol out of the fat that you eat. Cholesterol is the building material for the fatty gunk that closes down your blood vessels and irritates the lining of your vascular system, making clots more likely. Clots and narrow blood vessels eventually give rise to blockages and death of brain tissue, and even before that the oxygen supply is being limited. You don't want that. Insoluble fibre is meant to make you feel less hungry for longer, but even when that does not work, at least it keeps your bowels healthy if you take lots of water with it, and it will help you lose weight as part of a healthy lifestyle. (To be honest, even a buttered bread roll filled with chips could help as part of a healthy lifestyle. The secret is portion control.)

My dad hurt his back and had to take some painkillers. They made him constipated and his bowels got blocked. We did not realise what was happening but he ended up in great pain and it turned out he had not passed water for ten hours. He was retaining urine and had to have a catheter in to empty his bladder. Because he did not drink enough and the catheter was not kept clean he got a urine infection. By the time I got to the house you could smell the pee from the front door and he was roaring in pain and confusion. He went from mildly demented to completely mad in three days. (Daughter of Roger, 82)

- We do need some fat, but too much can lead to high

cholesterol. It is good to avoid artificial stuff called 'trans fat', which is oil that has been commercially hardened and used for frying or for processed foods. You get it a lot in commercial biscuits, cakes and pastries. There is naturally occurring trans fat, but it is in small quantities in any foods like meat or dairy so it is not so harmful. Use liquid oil for frying at home and avoid commercially fried foods. Saturated fats are found in fatty meat, butter and lard, sausages and pies, cheese and cream, and some commercial savoury snacks and chocolate. In the UK we eat too much of these; apart from narrowing the blood vessels it makes us fat. There is a direct relationship between being fat and dementia.

● Using unsaturated fat instead of saturated or trans fats can help lower blood cholesterol. You find it in oily fish, nuts and seeds, avocados and in sunflower and olive oils. You can also reduce the amount of fat by the cooking methods that you use, using less 'fast food' and checking the labels on tins and packets.

● Oily fish is rich in omega 3. I once suggested that this is good for the brain in a newspaper interview and got an angry letter from a scientist saying that there was not strong enough evidence of dementia-related benefits from omega 3 for him to be persuaded to change his diet on my recommendation. In truth, some studies say yes and some say no. Everyone's granny used to call fish 'brain food'. But it has been suggested that if you eat too much fish containing contaminants such as dioxins and polychlorinated biphenyls (PCBs)* you will make yourself

---

* The Food Standards Agency has pointed out that these chemicals pollute our waters and are concentrated in the fat stores of fish, so it recommends that adults should eat at least two but no more than four portions of fish a week, and vary the species. Potentially childbearing women and girls have lower limits.

ill, so it's recommended for adults that you limit yourself to four portions a week. Omega 3 has been described as anti-atherogenic, anti-inflammatory, antioxidant, anti-amyloid, neuroprotective (these words mean basically that it stops your blood vessels laying down fat and it stops the sort of brain damage that comes from fatty deposits and inflammation of the brain). Is this a wonder food? The research shows that omega 3 is associated with better brain health without actually proving that it causes better brain health. Researchers say that more research is needed. They would, wouldn't they?

- The danger of salt for your heart is well known, but studies have shown that older people who take too much salt and not enough exercise have reduced cognitive power. A teaspoon full a day is too much. When taste buds are dulled by age there is a temptation to lash on the salt to get some savour, but that's a bad idea.

- Cups of green tea apparently have the same chemicals that are in red wine that block the formation of clumps in the brain in Alzheimer's. There is also a suggestion from the research that a cup of coffee can make a positive difference in some people.

Vitamins

My uncle is a retired GP and every morning he takes a folic acid tablet, walks to the shop for his paper and then does the crossword, and says, 'Right, that's me without dementia for another day!' (Charlotte, talking about John, 79)

- Studies have shown that lower vitamin D concentrations in the blood are associated with poorer cognitive function and a higher risk of Alzheimer's disease. You can get it from food, but even in our misty islands we get most of our vitamin D from exposure to sunlight, which allows us to manufacture it ourselves. You'd have to eat a lot of oily fish or take a supplement to get the equivalent of ten minutes in the sunshine. It is also in eggs, and some margarine-type spreads are fortified with it, as are some breakfast cereals. But sunlight is best, particularly in the summer months, when the rays are the right wavelength. Lots of people with dementia, particularly in care homes, never get outside at all. That's not clever.

- There has been research where people with MCI took very large quantities of vitamin B and it seemed to slow down their decline, and fewer of them went on to develop dementia. You'd need to take those vitamins in such large quantities that you'd be best to ask your doctor before embarking on this too enthusiastically. People with a low blood level of folic acid (which is part of the B complex of vitamins) can have dementia-like symptoms and that is why your GP should test you for this if you complain about your memory.

Mental stimulation

If you don't use it, you lose it! Learning something new is good for your brain. It is like a 'keep fit' regime would be for your heart. The more you use your brain, the better it is for you. You develop a sort of spare capacity that will stand you in good stead if some of your brain tissue starts to shrink or fails because the blood supply has been compromised. Brain scans of people who have learned a lot about something – for example, London taxi drivers who have to memorise street names and routes – show a real physical increase in the amount of brain tissue that they have. If you have more brain capacity, you can resist the effects of loss of brain cells for longer.

- Enjoy games and puzzles that make you think. Sudoku is very popular for those of us who can't do crossword puzzles. The newsagent always has stacks of word-search puzzle books and you can buy brain-training programs to run on your PC or Game Boy. These are so much fun they can end up being mildly addictive. The research on this is variable (just like most of the research). Some people think that if you practise this sort of thing, the main effect is that you get better at the specific puzzle, rather than improving your total brain power, but others are firmly convinced of the benefits. Companies have been sued for claiming that their brain-training game prevented dementia, which shows that it is possible to exaggerate the benefits.

- Vary your habits. Don't live life on automatic pilot, doing the same thing all the time. Challenge yourself with something new every day of your life. Explore, read, talk to people and find things out. If you develop dementia a whole lot of life will start to become challenging, so practise facing challenges now. Learn how to program your mobile phone, or Skype, or set the date and time on the answering machine. Go to town by a different route. Take evening classes.

Quality sleep

- Good sleep seems to predispose to the delay of dementia symptoms, and dementia itself is unspeakably tiring, for both the person with dementia and carers. So a good sleep schedule is vital. Improving sleep is not listed in the World Health Organization guidelines on risk reduction, but it is clear that there is some association between sleep disorders and dementia for which more research is needed.

- Chapter 9 has ideas on how you can make the bedroom the best it can be for inducing sleep by making simple design changes and using easily available technology, while Chapter 8 has some strategies for managing nocturnal wandering.

- Sleep is influenced by a hormone in your body called melatonin. It sets the body clock. Blood levels are lower in older people and even lower in people with dementia. You can stimulate the metabolism of melatonin by exposing your eyes to daylight, especially in the morning. If you want to sleep tonight, get lots of daylight today. The melatonin slows down bodily functions at night and makes you sleepy. These are two sleep-related reasons for going for a walk in daylight: one is to make you physically tired and the other is to set your body clock with melatonin so that you go to sleep at the same time as most other people where you live. The vitamin D production is a bonus, because it helps reduce falls, apart from any cognitive benefits it brings.

- Smart napping: there is a phenomenon called 'sun-downing' when the person with dementia starts to get irritable and restless in the late afternoon. It has been speculated that this is related to changes in the light level, but more people now think that it is really mainly caused by fatigue, so an afternoon nap might be a good idea. Getting the balance of being busy and having rests is easier if you know the person.

Mum always did a lot of housework, and now when we don't know what to do, we find some housework for her to do. She polishes brass, irons shirts, cleans floors. Of course she is slow and not very accurate, but it keeps her calm and busy. She sleeps better at night when she's been busy. (Daughter of Janice, 62)

Stress management and daily relaxation

No one can get inner peace by pouncing on it. (Harry E. Fosdick, American pastor)

- Stress can make you look as if you have dementia when

you don't. If you have MCI stress can make your symptoms worse. If you have the underlying disease in your brain that causes dementia you might not have any symptoms at all, until stress brings them out. Stress is very, very bad for people with dementia. The stress can make the symptoms so bad that the person may not be able to cope at home. Reducing stress reduces the need for medication.

- Practise breathing. Breathing seems so very simple. You inhale and exhale, taking in oxygen and getting rid of carbon dioxide. Your body is really clever and regulates the speed of breathing according to how much oxygen your muscles and other organs need. After running up the stairs you automatically speed up. Hyperventilation is when you breathe faster than your body needs, and it is almost exclusively caused by tension and worry. Other breathing problems occur when you take lots of little inhalations that don't fill your lungs. The fresh air doesn't get as far as the deep pockets of your lungs, where the exchange of oxygen happens. You take lots of shallow breaths without getting much of the precious stuff into your bloodstream. Most of your bodily functions work automatically and you can't control them. It's hard to slow your heartbeat by thinking about it, and you can't consciously regulate how fast urine is made. But you can take charge of your breathing. Slower breathing can lead to relaxation. We all know that, but there's science and body chemistry behind it. Walking slowly can lead to deeper and slower breathing, so a slow walk can help relaxation, and relaxation exercises often focus on tensing and relaxing muscles in turn while controlling breathing. There's evidence of how this helps with a wide range of health care issues, from diabetes to muscle strains.

- You can learn a range of relaxation techniques and find one that suits you. You may have tried yoga or t'ai chi, but there are some that don't need classroom instruction. 'Mindfulness' is the ability to remain aware of how you are feeling right now. You don't think about the past or worry about the future. By staying calm and in the moment, you can reduce the feelings of stress that might overwhelm you. Sit comfortably and focus on an object in your surroundings or close your eyes. 'Visualisation' is when you close your eyes and imagine a restful scene and then explore it in huge detail, imagining all the sensory experiences you are having in that scene, including sound and touch. You can learn how to use these techniques on your own and they are practical for a busy person to undertake in their own home. Look for apps, audiobooks and books that you can buy or find information online. NHS Stress Busters has advice on the NHS Choices website (www.nhs.uk).

● Religious observance is of crucial importance to some people but may become harder to continue in the circumstances that come with dementia and caring. Having a religious belief is associated with lower stress levels, and it is clear that engaging in familiar and safe practices like singing and attending worship can give great comfort. There is further research to be done on whether religious belief has a positive effect on health, but it is clear that for many people, including caregivers, an opportunity to practise their faith is vital. How dementia is 'framed' or perceived in the mind of any human is shaped by their attitude to life, personality, their belief in a soul, or personhood ... and knowing how someone perceives this is very important for understanding how to reduce their stress. Dementia might be perceived as a punishment from a deity for some previous sin or wickedness, or accepted as something to be borne on a journey to paradise. How people think of death and dying matters in this space and benefit or damage can occur depending on how we respond to the spiritual or religious needs of the person. You may be the Jewish lady singing Christian hymns to comfort a lady with dementia (www.youtube.com/watch?v=_ chOko4TFaM) or you may be an atheist reassuring someone that their god will not forget them. When you are caring for someone with a belief, what you yourself believe almost doesn't matter.

Malcolm Goldsmith, a priest with an interest in dementia, wrote *In a Strange Land* in 2004, which is still the finest book on dementia and religious faith. He examines questions from a Christian perspective. People ask, 'Why me? Is this God's punishment?' They wrestle with ethical issues about the belief systems of those giving care: 'As a doctor, can I pray with my patient?' Malcolm offers practical and supportive answers. Here I first read about the American nun Sister Laura. She feared that she was going to forget Jesus because of dementia, and she said to the founding investigator of the Nun Study (a study to examine predictors of Alzheimer's disease in a homogenous group), David Snowdon, 'I finally realised that I may not remember Him, but He will remember me.'

All religions respect older people. The Quran recognises the effect of dementia in older people. It speaks of how some are 'sent back to a feeble age, so that they know nothing after having known much' and tells us that we must be kind to parents, and 'say not to them a word of contempt, nor repel them, but address them in terms of honour ... even as they cherished me in childhood'. Caring for your ageing parents is incumbent on Muslims. The role of religion in dementia care, and in making people contented is very important in very many faiths.

Active social life

● Volunteer! There are so many reasons for volunteering that it deserves a book of its own. Making a difference to other people, having fun, keeping up your skills, making friends … and you can learn new things. People once thought of volunteers as 'do-gooders' who help other people by giving of themselves for no reward. In fact you can't escape the reward, even if you won't take any money for what you do. You are not filling a gap left by someone else who ought to be doing this, you are giving something extra that makes a difference, something that would not be possible without you. Be sure to work for an organisation that offers proper induction and supervision, and ask about expenses. You've got skills that you can pass on. How many young people can you teach to bake, or to run a decent allotment, or to keep chickens?

There is such a fashion for keeping chickens now. They do evening classes and sell books on the subject. We always had chickens when I was a girl, and it has been great fun buying some and showing the grandchildren how to make a bit of money selling eggs. They are amazed at what I know. (Anne, Birmingham)

● Join a club. If you pick the right club you can indulge in your interest. If you are boring your family and friends to death with your knowledge of steam engines, imagine the pleasure of being with others who will talk about it until long after everyone else has ceased to be interested. Bliss. Socialising is good for delaying dementia symptoms and reducing them. No one is sure why, but who cares if it means you get to see newly discovered pictures of the Flying Scotsman? A book club will encourage you to read books that you would not normally choose, and even if you are only listening to others discussing the issues that arise from the books it can stimulate your thinking. The issues in a good book are universal and eternal and you can join in a discussion of those issues from your life experience, even if your recent memories are a bit hazy.

- Taking classes is a good idea, even though it is often said that people with dementia can't learn new things. You can live in the moment, enjoying the experience, without having to worry about tests and exams. An example is a class run in Melbourne, Australia, by the National Gallery of Victoria, that is specifically for people with dementia. The programme has been developed to tap into the imagination of people with dementia through multiple workshops and visits to the gallery. Many museums and galleries in the UK offer similar projects. Art triggers both the mind and the emotions and, of course, if you take lots of classes before you get dementia, it can delay the onset. Education, brain training … call it what you like. It is probably the social aspect that makes the biggest difference. Anyone going to the pub later?

- Keeping connected with family and friends offers great health benefits. It could be that just keeping tabs on them is a significant mental exercise that keeps the grey matter active.

We've got two children and six grandchildren and one great-granddaughter, and one is retired and three are working, and we've had two weddings in the last five years. And the new baby. And the grandchildren are working in England and New Zealand, so we have to write to them and talk on the phone. The grandson lost his job … he was really worried for a while, so we kept phoning him … [Laughs] It's a full-time job just remembering the birthday cards, never mind everything else! I have to keep a book and mark it all on the calendar. (Grandmother, 85)

● Some people don't have big families and rely even more on friends. You need to make dates and get out and keep seeing them as much as you can. Research shows that the stimulation you get does not have to be as highbrow as doing the crossword in *The Times*. Ladies who go to bingo (a much-maligned simple betting game) are in better cognitive shape than those who stay at home. The complexities of organising your bus, your pals, the money and just getting there are a challenge in themselves, never mind keeping an eye on the numbers. The best socialising is whatever you enjoy most, because that is what you will keep up, and it is persevering that makes a difference.

Sensory impairment is a real issue. If you have hearing loss and it is not corrected it can double your chance of having dementia, so ask your GP or go to one of the high-street practitioners in an optician or pharmacy and get a hearing test. Excellent quality hearing aids are available on the NHS, and other more fashionable models privately.

Is there a miracle cure?

When you surf the net looking for ideas about what makes a difference in dementia, there is a lot of information out there. There have been stories about coconut oil and turmeric, ginkgo biloba and vitamin supplements, cow's milk colostrum and eating pansies, and a whole range of nutritional advice that is supposed to improve brain function. My problem with all of these is that they may send people off on a wild-goose chase. The stressed and anxious buyer under pressure will spend money that they can't afford on things whose benefits are not proven, with side effects they were not warned about. They are not helped by the way in which research is undertaken and how it is reported in sensational terms in the media. From day to day 'miracles' are celebrated and then disproved. It is hard at times to know what to do for the best, because at some point it might be discovered that one of these really works.

However, there is no escaping the fact that at the moment the intervention for which there is the greatest evidence of effectiveness is exercise, along with socialising and keeping active in any way that you can.

Chapter 7

Managing care at home

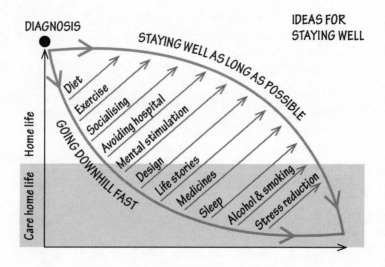

IDEAS FOR
STAYING WELL

DIAGNOSIS

STAYING WELL AS LONG AS POSSIBLE

IDEAS FOR
STAYING WELL

GOING DOWNHILL FAST

Home life

Care home life

Diet

Exercise

Socialising

Avoiding hospital

Mental stimulation

Design

Life stories

Medicines

Sleep

Alcohol & smoking

Stress reduction

Can you stay at home for ever?

Most people with dementia live at home and half of those who live in their own home live alone. It is perfectly possible for a person with dementia to be happy at home for a long time and to do very well, right to the end of life. However, some people reach a stage where they need to be looked after more intensively. Dementia is a long-term condition that gradually worsens, but many people with dementia become ill and die of something else before the symptoms get too serious, so it's important to plan for living well and not feel that everything has suddenly shuddered to a halt the day the diagnosis is given. This chapter gives some help in understanding how to make care at home work.

My dad started to lose some of his words and reached the point where he could not spell his own name. But we travelled and walked and worked in the garden right up till the day he had his heart attack and died. (Daughter of 67-year-old man with early-onset dementia)

There are three major elements to this – staying in the right place, keeping well through a healthy diet, and making life easier through design features in the home. Attention to those things that will make the person feel secure and relaxed can help to ensure that staying at home is a good option.

In general people want to put off as long as possible the time when they might have to give up their own home to go to other accommodation. Good care homes and nursing homes are in despair because of bad publicity about a small number of really unsatisfactory care homes. The good ones provide charming and comfortable places for people to live in at a difficult time of life; but calamitous stories dominate the press and public imagination. That shapes the perception of families and friends when they are considering moving someone into a care home. Many people at the early stages of dementia are quite clear that they want to stay at home for ever. We all love our homes. You spend your whole life getting it just the way you want it, so why would you leave it and go somewhere else, particularly when you're not feeling right? In this chapter there are ideas about how to stay at home for as long as possible. But there is a postscript reminding you that if you do move to a care home or nursing home it is not a sign of failure or betrayal. A day may come when you think it is right for such a move. You can be kind to your family by telling them that when the day comes, even if you are not well enough to take part in the decision, you accept that this is what they may have to do for you. You need to trust someone else to do what is best for you and that is why choosing the right person to have power of attorney is so important (see Chapter 13).

In the beginning: preparation and enjoying life to the full

Getting used to the idea of what dementia really means takes time. Everyone is different. Some people want to tell everyone immediately, while others need a bit of thinking time. It is possible that there has been a lot of worry about what was going wrong and at least now you have a name to put to it. If you've had experience of someone with dementia in the family before, it is worth getting up-to-date information because a lot has changed in recent years.

My grandmother had it, and there were no pills, and it was the sort of thing you kept secret. They just said 'she's senile' and we all looked the other way until it fell apart in her house and we got her into hospital. Then she went in a home. (Andrew, 55)

Dementia has been high up on government health agendas in all developed countries in recent years. In every case, health department policies have been driving doctors to make a diagnosis earlier and earlier. This means that when you learn that dementia is the problem there will still be a whole lot of living to do before life gets really tough. This is precious time during which you can enjoy your home and your home life. Even if the person with dementia does not live with you, there are things that you can do together to make preparation for the future. If you are affected by dementia yourself, you can do things to keep yourself well and happy for as long as possible.

Advance preparations

You may be wondering about whether to move house. In general staying put is a good idea for people with dementia. Moving to a new location can be harrowing for any of us. It takes a lot of planning and physical energy and there is the worry about mortgages, tenancy agreements or leases, how much it costs and whether it is the right thing to do. If the motivation is something wonderful like a new garden, more space or a new job it can be brilliant. However, if you are not feeling well and the move is not for a positive reason, it could be traumatic, especially if it feels like putting one foot in the grave. A person with dementia might feel coerced into it.

I want Dad to move to be near us because he is getting dementia and I want to look after him. He wants to stay put but that's not an option. I've told him. (Mrs B., 60, daughter with power of attorney for her father)

Nevertheless, not everyone wants to stay on their own. If you have been widowed, and live by yourself, you may feel lonely and isolated even if you do have help from social services. You may decide to move nearer family, whether that is in their home, in special housing where you can get assistance, or just in another house or flat nearby. If you are going to have to move there are design issues about the new place which you should consider (see Chapter 9) and it is best to make the move while you are feeling physically healthy. If it is inevitable, then it's best to move in a controlled way, rather than as a result of an emergency.

Davinia had a fall at home and went into hospital, so I gave up the house and when she came out I moved her straight into the new place. (Nephew of a woman with dementia)

Everything works better when we feel we have some choice and control, and this is as true for a person with dementia as for anyone else. It's helpful to minimise the number of moves that a person with dementia has to make, because each move is stressful and increasing stress often makes dementia symptoms worse. Having to learn a new environment is particularly difficult for a person with dementia. Planning is really important, to iron out as many details of the move as possible in advance.

There is a clear and growing need for services which are available shortly after diagnosis and which focus expressly on helping someone to carry on living independently in their own home. There are lots of models of this and the main issue is whether there is one near you. The health or social care staff that you meet, or the local voluntary organisation such as the Alzheimer's Society or Age UK, may be able to help you to find out about them.

One of the determining factors will be finance. If you had a social services assessment at the earliest stage it may be that you don't yet qualify for much support, because it depends on your level of need as well as your finances (see Chapter 10). In Scotland there is a guarantee of one year's post-diagnostic support from the health and social care system, but that is not financial. It is more focused on information about your options and 'signposting'. Some local authorities and voluntary organisations will do a 'wealth check' for you to help you work out whether you are getting all the allowances to which you are entitled. If you want to stay at home and you suspect that you will not be eligible for social services support as a result of a means test, it may be worth talking to an independent financial adviser about how to manage the cost of your future care needs.

Staying at home is made possible by a range of interventions, some of which cost money. It is important not to worry about the money but do something about it. We are fortunate in the UK in the extent to which there is a safety net for people who don't have capital. Chapter 10 will give you some idea of how to find out what is available to you from the social care system. There are also supports which can be given to you through voluntary organisations.

In Chapter 13 you will see that the powers of attorney can focus on financial or welfare issues, and this is a good time to talk to your chosen attorney about what you want for the future. They will have to decide on your behalf if you can't decide in future, but you need to make sure that they understand your thinking while you are still able to tell them.

What are the options for housing?

Housing will play an increasingly important role in improving the world for people with dementia. Delaying the need for residential care is a major part of controlling the cost of dementia. If the home setting is good, it could shorten the length of stay when someone is admitted to hospital and help to prevent them having to go from there to a care home. There are many examples of good practice from housing associations and home improvement agencies that provide specialist housing, adaptations for your own house and a range of flexible support.

The number of people living with dementia is set to rise to over one million. The majority of these people will live in the community, in their own homes, and they want to stay there for as long as possible.

Early intervention services centred on people's homes have the greatest potential to improve the quality of life of people with dementia and their carers. (Alistair Burns, National Clinical Director for Dementia for England)

The concept of a tailored design of house or apartment for a person with dementia has been around since the 1980s. This not only concerns the design of the residence and the use of assistive technology, but also embraces the idea of staff who are trained to come and give support to you in that setting, while allowing you to live independently for as long as possible. When looking for this sort of place you will find it called 'housing with care', 'extra care housing', 'assisted living' and 'continuing-care housing'. These schemes may be for generalised groups of retired people and sometimes the management or the other residents are not very tolerant of people with dementia. In many cases they are operated by non-profit housing associations, but businesses are also seizing opportunities to provide for this market.

Retirement villages and complexes

A retirement village was traditionally a housing complex designed for older people who care for themselves, but increasingly the estate on which the housing is built has other levels of supported accommodation to which the residents can move when their needs increase over time. The idea of owning a place in a private retirement village may appeal to those who have the means to buy the apartment, studio flat or house and pay the maintenance or service charges. This typically would offer the comfort of a luxury high-specification cottage or apartment and a range of facilities in a secluded environment. People can move into the community when they are over the age of fifty-five and undergo transition to an onsite care home if that is subsequently required. In the USA they might have 100,000 residents. Not exactly a village, then. The UK versions are more modest in size. You may prefer to live in a smaller complex, which could be a block of retirement flats or a small scheme of ground-level houses in a mixed area such as a real town or village, so that you see and meet people of different ages and can access facilities that everyone else uses.

Although the village looked great, we really needed to have a think about all the questions. Could I bring my own furniture and was my dog allowed to come? Was there any control over the service charges? It turned out that there was something called an 'assignment fee' that I had to consider. I needed to get my lawyer to advise me. Then it turned out that they wanted a report from my doctor as well that I was in 'good health'. I decided against that one. (M., 72)

Funding such a move may be prohibitive for many. If you are already a homeowner over fifty-five you can use 'equity release', which is a method where you use the money locked up in the value of your own home to buy a retirement home. A service charge is levied to cover maintenance costs, security and a warden, lounges and other shared areas. You would also be able to buy in personal and domestic services, so you need to budget for that as well. The advantage is that you are independent and have some control over your circumstances. You need independent legal and financial advice for all of this.

Living with relatives

Living with relatives can be wonderful. A multigenerational family can have lots of fun. Of course there are areas of stress too, as when any family members choose to live together. If young people move back home to live with parents, rules and boundaries can be set to avoid conflicts, but for a person with dementia, a condition that changes, it is difficult to make hard and fast rules.

However, there are some simple strategies that you can adopt – for example, having certain rooms, such as the bedroom, that are private, and knocking before entering. If you've taken in a parent or moved in with them, don't take all their chores and activities off them. Keeping on doing things is good for a person with dementia. You need to be clear about compensation and what the financial arrangements will be. That is simpler if you have power of attorney, but even so, it's a good idea to keep the rest of the family informed about what is happening in case of misunderstandings. If you set goals and clearly communicate plans it will prevent some potential battles.

My mother moved in with us, and this is the best move we ever made. She loves the children and they can spend so much time with her. When she shuts the door on her part of the house at night, she is completely private, but she could call us if she needed us. She's in the early stage of dementia and we know we might have to rethink one day, but we are fine at present. (Janice, daughter of M., 72)

Or you could stay where you are. If you've lived there for a long time, lapses in recent memory are not so serious, because you'd still find your way home.

Local authority or housing association supported or sheltered housing

Many local authorities have sheltered housing, mainly one-bedroom homes, which are adapted for people with particular needs or disabilities. The houses may have a built-in alarm system, including monitoring of activity in many cases. Some have community rooms, laundry facilities or guest rooms for use by families. In some cases meals are also provided and that is sometimes called 'very sheltered housing'. In addition to the weekly rent for your house, you will probably pay a service charge, which covers the cost of the alarm system and responses and any agreed housing support. A housing support officer is usually available to help you complete any forms, in particular if you have a low income and are eligible for housing benefit. When you move in, a support worker is allocated to you and they assess what support you will need. This could include help to attend appointments or social activities, and help with managing your mail or paying bills, etc.

Staying at home with Live-in Care or House sharing

If you wish to stay in your own home and your care needs increase, you may consider live-in care as an alternative to a care home. It depends on your resources, and this is not affordable for everyone. A home owner might decide to remortgage their home and use that asset to pay for live-in care. The fees are roughly equivalent to staying in a high-end care home, but you would still have to pay the cost of running your home, such as fuel, council tax and other household expenses on top of the fee.

We provide round-the-clock care for two weeks at a time, then swap with a woman who covers the following two weeks. Each day we get two hours free to get out and about, and if the client is poorly an agency can cover that, but often they are well enough to manage alone for those two hours if you time it right – for example, having an afternoon nap. It is usually very comfortable living in the spare room and we do all the cooking, cleaning and shopping as well as taking the client out and about, and entertaining them at home. It is a real pleasure. (Quote from a couple who provide live-in care)

Another option is house sharing, where a lodger comes to stay and pays part or all of their 'rent' in the form of personal care and support, on a very part-time basis. It is reassuring for the client to have someone else staying there, and it can help with housing needs for the lodger. Doing this through an agency provides protection such as reference checks, etc., and making sure that legal issues such as tenancy rights are observed.

Maintaining a healthy diet: keeping well – for everyone

The more fit and well you feel, whether you are a person with dementia or a carer, the better you will be able to handle the unexpected situations and stresses that arise which could, if handled badly, lead to the person with dementia having to give up their home. There is more advice in Chapter 3 for carers on how to stay well.

Eating and drinking properly can make a lot of difference. Keeping a healthy diet going can be challenging at the best of times, but it is really important to maintain the strength and health of everyone in the house by making sure of regular meals. If this is difficult, you should be assessed by social services for a meal delivery service. You may have to pay towards that. There are private companies that deliver meals direct, often the same company that supplies the local authority. You might go out more for meals, because that is not necessarily overly expensive.

*We go to the supermarket café every day for lunch. We don't need
a lot so we have the 'kid's meal' (they laugh when they give me
the colouring book, but I save them up for the grandchildren). It's
good to have a cooked meal once a day and I don't have to do all the
preparation and wash up. It gets us out, and I see a lot of the same
people there each day. The ladies at the till are getting to know us. It
is much cheaper than the meals on wheels because we can choose what
we fancy each day and nothing gets wasted or thrown away. (D., 83)*

Many women of an older generation relied on their husbands
for driving and if he is the person with dementia the transport
problems can be considerable. For food shopping, consider using
the online shopping and delivery service from a supermarket. If
you are not confident with that, you may have someone in the
family who will help you and in some areas the local authority
or a voluntary organisation provides a low-cost shopping service.

*I know one lady in Northumberland with a daughter in Canada
who does her weekly shop for the mum online, and it gets delivered
as regular as clockwork. That's very good, but we have set up a local
social enterprise and we do it using volunteers for people who don't
have families. (Community worker)*

While on the subject of eating and drinking, staying hydrated is
really important. It is not unusual for older people to selectively
avoid drinking in order to try to reduce the need to go to the
toilet. This is not clever. You need water for all your bodily functions, including your blood supply, and if you allow yourself to
get dry you will lose some of your cognitive functions. If you've
already got some dementia symptoms, dehydration will make
the situation worse. You will get confused. It is also very likely
that you will develop a urinary tract infection (sometimes called
an UTI) and get even more confused as a result. You can end

up in hospital just from not drinking enough water, and this is particularly true if you are already coming down with dementia. Keep your pee a nice pale straw colour. If it gets any darker drink more. If it gets smelly see a doctor as fast as you can to get antibiotics before you end up in an ambulance. Water is the stuff of life. So drink some. Tea is also good. In fact almost any fluid helps, and you get fluid from other food, like soups and custard.

Complications around eating and drinking

At times it can be more difficult to get someone with dementia to take the right amount of the right food. This section is about the practical issues involved with getting them to eat, even if they don't seem to have much appetite for food.

Eating and drinking are essential for life, and a source of great pleasure for most of us. As outlined before, a person with dementia might begin to have difficulty with shopping and cooking food by themselves, and when that happens their diet can suffer. But as time goes by their dementia might mean they find it difficult to recognise and enjoy food, and so they will require help to make sure they have a good diet. Practical things can be done to make it more likely that people with dementia will continue to enjoy their food for as long as possible and get the benefit of a good diet and fluids.

There is a current fad for a slimming diet (5:2) that involves eating only a small amount of calories over twenty-four hours twice a week. Even if you take a normal diet on the other five days you will lose weight. If a person with dementia misses eating properly on only two days in the week, it is as if they are on this slimming regime. It is no surprise that under these circumstances they will lose weight at a time in life when that is not desirable for most people.

Drinking

In any emergency lack of fluid is always more serious than lack of food. A young, healthy and fit person can survive without fluid for a few days, and without food for a few weeks, but they'll not be very well.

Not having enough to drink can cause deterioration in a person with dementia much more quickly. The brain ceases to work well in anyone who is dehydrated at any age. Children in schools in the past were never offered fluids during classes, but it is recognised now that they learn better if they have open access to drinking water. For someone with dementia who is already struggling with their thinking, not having enough to drink can quickly make them more confused.

How much is needed depends on the person's metabolism and their activity, and the temperature in which they are living, set by the heating in their home or the weather outside. You can tell if the person has not had enough to drink usually from their urine becoming dark and concentrated, and from their skin losing its flexibility. People can die of dehydration very fast, like someone who exercises in the sun, or a baby locked in a hot car. A person with dementia who is dehydrating over a matter of days will have sunken eyes and a dry mouth. The heartbeat becomes more rapid and the person lethargic. It's very serious.

The person is more likely to drink if there are lots of cues. Have the kettle and teapot in full view along with the tea bags. If you have a glass-fronted fridge, have lots of attractive bottles of juice on show. Keep jugs of water and glasses somewhere convenient. Suggest 'a cuppa' at every opportunity. Have drinks on the table at mealtimes. Just reminding the person to drink has great value. Suggest having a drink every time you talk to the person with dementia.

Junior doctors in hospitals should carry a glass of water and offer a sip to the patient in between questions when interviewing them. The nurses are so busy and the person has so little support to stay hydrated. It is the least they can do. (Hospital consultant)

Dehydration in hospital is very common for practical reasons. If the person staying at home is allowed to get dehydrated, the danger is that they will end up in a hospital that only makes the situation worse for them.

What should people drink? In general anything is better than nothing, but of course water is very good. For younger people water is best, but for older people in particular, if their appetite is poor, you have to be sure that you are not filling them up with so much water that they can't eat enough. Make sure in those cases that they are drinking things that offer calories and vitamins – for example, a milkshake or fresh fruit juice. Tea and coffee with caffeine in them might be limited towards the end of the day if you want to reduce nocturnal wandering, but they are great first thing in the morning when people wake up. If the person has blood pressure problems, then they may have to have decaffeinated drinks. The amount of fluid needed depends on what you are doing and how hot the environment is. Hospitals can get very hot, even if you are sitting still all the time. Alcohol can be nice, but you need to be sure that it is not interfering with medication, so get approval first from the doctor and remember that the smaller and older you are, the less you can tolerate alcohol. Used in excess it also causes dehydration.

Going to the toilet can be complicated at times, and it is not unusual for people with dementia to deliberately reduce their fluid intake to avoid the complication of having to find the loo in a hurry. The problem with this is that it will lead to some increase in their dementia symptoms, and if they do it long enough they will get a urinary tract infection, or a 'chill on the bladder', that will cause even more confusion and can lead to a hospital admission for intravenous antibiotics, as we have already seen. It is a shame to end up on a 'drip' because you were trying to avoid wetting yourself. If continence is an issue, people need to be directed to the continence nurse via the GP to get assessment and support, and discreet pads if needed. It should not be a problem that leads to people avoiding fluids.

Take particular care when the person with dementia goes into hospital or a care home.

When my mum was in hospital they put her water jug where she could not reach it. She could not even see it, of course, because it was clear, and the water was clear and so was the glass. I put it within her reach and put a bit of orange cordial in it, and she helped herself after that. (Jane, daughter of D., 85)

Eating

We were always taught that dementia was a wasting disease … people lost weight rapidly in the old psychiatric hospital before they died. (Dementia nurse)

It was not necessary in most cases for those people to lose weight. Of course, towards the very end of life, as the body closes down and the person is dying, there is a natural process that takes place, but people with dementia in the past were quite simply not fed properly in institutions. Learning from what went wrong then can give us a clue about how to do it properly at home. The power you have when the person is in their own home means that you can avoid these hazards.

The problems included:

- rigid mealtimes that came and went whether you were hungry or not;

- no choice over what was served or influence over the menu;
- food served in uncomfortable surroundings and in unattractive servings;
- too much or too little served on the plate;
- more than one course stacked on the tray or table at the same time;
- nothing to eat between meals;
- a long fast from 'tea' at 5.30 p.m. until breakfast at 8 a.m.;
- no allowances made for the changes in dementia;
- no allowances made for sensory and physical impairments;
- hurried shovelling of food into people who needed help to eat;
- use of sedation, so people were too drowsy to eat;
- uneaten food removed without keeping a record, or weighing the person regularly.

At home you can make sure that all of these problems are avoided. Eating away from home also carries memories of all sorts of complicated things, like how to pay and how to behave in front of others, which can be confusing and cause distress. Care homes are getting better at managing the problem.

We could not work out why Florence would not eat in the care home. When I sat with her she eventually whispered, 'I've got no money … I'm not able to pay for this.' She thought she was in a restaurant or hotel and because they had taken away her handbag she thought she was going to be embarrassed by a bill. At every mealtime we got into the habit of discreetly letting her know that it was all paid for in advance and she could take as much as she wanted. (Care worker)

Mealtimes

The person with dementia may not wish to eat when it is 'time to eat'. Some prefer to graze throughout the day, never actually wanting to sit down at a table.

I keep a cookie jar and bowls of sweets around the place all the time, as well as bananas and nice soft fruit like strawberries. I see Mum just going up and helping herself. I've got a fridge with wrapped tiny sandwiches and savouries that I can produce at a moment's notice if she fancies one. (Daughter of 76-year-old woman with dementia)

Food should be available at any time, night or day. You can make this possible in your own home in simple practical ways. Traditionally there have been limitations to when food may be available in hospitals and care homes, and the tyranny of food hygiene control has at times meant that people have been starving in those settings because the risk of food poisoning was overestimated.

We used to give them scrambled eggs in the evening if patients were peckish, but they stopped that because of fear of salmonella. (Nurse)

If the person eats well at home, you need to investigate whether you can supply them with food for snacking if you have to temporarily leave them in a hospital or care home.

If for important reasons you would like the person to eat at a particular time – for example, because that is the only time you are available to support them by cooking or assisting them to eat – there are practical things that can help.

- Cue the fact that it is time to eat by creating smells of cooking artificially or naturally. Machines that emit appetite-stimulating smells are available commercially, or perhaps this can happen in the ordinary way through cooking and maybe involving the person with dementia in the cooking. Preparing a meal can make you hungry. Fried-onion smells will make people buy hot dogs that taste of virtually nothing, so use cooking onions as an appetite stimulant for your nourishing meals. The smell of vanilla or of baking bread are famously mouthwatering. The smell of toasting fruit bread is said to be particularly appetising and likewise Bakewell tart.

- If eating at a table is what the person prefers set the table formally and make it attractive, using napkins and cruets, then get them to sit up at the table on a comfortable chair. Other people prefer a tray on their lap ... everyone is different and you need to do what works.

- Use contrasting crockery so that the food can be seen on the plate and stands out from the tabletop, tray or tablecloth. A portion of white mash with white fish, on a white plate with a white tablecloth, may be almost invisible to a person with depth perception problems and ageing eyes.

- Reduce distractions by switching off the radio and television, and focusing on the food. Make sure there is lots of light on the food.

- Eat with the person with dementia. Eating is a social activity.

Mealtimes that are pleasant help with good digestion. Taking time is also important.

Dr Kevin Charras in research in a care home introduced a very long lunchtime where everyone took about three hours to eat a number of courses. Everyone put on weight. What was the point of rushing? There was little else to do. (Report from J.M. on research from Fondation Médéric Alzheimer)

It may be more difficult to arrange this leisurely pace at home, so making sure that there are tempting snacks outside of meal times is important. Just think the opposite of what one does when trying to lose weight. Eat between meals. Have high-calorie snacks. Enjoy!

Choice

The simplest ideas are often the best. If you want someone to eat, offer them what they really, really like.

For days on end Dad only seemed to want to eat custard and bananas. Not a very balanced diet, and an odd thing to ask for first thing in the morning. He was not interested in eggs or cheese, or steak pies or all his usual favourite things. The community psychiatric nurse reassured me that I should just give him what he wanted in the meantime and only worry if it went on for weeks. In the end he started to refuse the custard and was asking for other things, and no harm seemed to come of it. I just felt a bit guilty. (Daughter of 70-year-old man)

It is important to stay calm and flexible about eating and drinking. If you are a member of the family or a friend you probably know what the person prefers to eat and drink, and when.

Common problems of ageing and stress

A general reduction in the sense of taste and smell in old people can become greater with dementia. People sometimes find it hard to have a family meal and eat alongside people with later stages of dementia if they are displaying behavioural problems at mealtimes, including playing with food, refusing to eat it or spitting it out. There may be several reasons for this.

I got to know with Mum that if she did not like something she'd just spit it back at me. I learned not to try new flavours or textures. Eventually it was as if she had forgotten how to eat, or chew or swallow. (Sarah, daughter of Alice, 92)

In other cases the person may become agitated and angry at mealtimes because of a combination of difficulties.

Gordon hated eating with other people. He felt as if he was being watched by them, and he hated the loss of dignity because we had to help him spoon his food to his mouth. With the Lewy body dementia he got a bit paranoid and at times he actually thought the food might be poisoned. (Alison, wife of Gordon, 68)

Trying to make mealtimes as enjoyable and stress-free as possible is an art. One important element is the place, and the accessibility of the table and chair. People who are eating in groups may feel under stress to complete their food at the same time as others, even if they are still a little bit hungry, so watch for that when eating out. Cutlery is available with different larger handles, for ease of use, and there are cups and mugs specifically designed to cope with practical problems in older people, such as the weight of the cup, the size and balance of the handle, and whether it is easy to grasp in two hands. Non-slip placemats can help prevent plates from moving around, and a plate with a lip on the edge can help prevent food from sliding off the plate altogether. But don't go overboard.

I hated seeing my mother being offered food on plastic plates. We've found some nice coloured pottery that meets her needs and we don't mind if it gets broken. Plastic is for babies and for picnics, not a hot dinner for a lady of eighty. (Sarah, daughter of Alice, 92)

Dementia changes

In some cases enjoyment of food decreases as the dementia increases. The person may seem to lose interest in eating and drinking. It is not just that they 'forget' to eat and drink. Their appetite might seem to be poor even if food is put in front of them. It is important to be aware of the sorts of problems that might arise and have some practical ideas about possible solutions. People get quite upset if they have prepared a meal and it is rejected. There is a lot of emotion attached to food.

If as a result of the dementia the person is taking less exercise, this can give rise to constipation, which will in turn reduce appetite. Make sure that plenty of fluids are taken and ensure that the diet includes fibre. The loss of appetite and constipation can be made worse by painkillers or the side effects of other medicines. Check with the doctor, nurse or pharmacist. When the person has dementia they might not tell you that they are in pain. For example, a poorly fitting denture or a sore mouth might not get mentioned to you, but the person just stops eating.

It is quite common for people with dementia to have depression in addition. Depression can reduce appetite. It is important to get it diagnosed and treated. Try to keep the person involved in choosing and preparing food to keep up interest and check that you are giving them 'a little of what they fancy'.

Familiarity and routine are important for a person with dementia, and so when planning meals you should take this into consideration. Some people with dementia pace around and use up a lot of energy, and in those cases you may want to enrich their diet in order to get enough calories into them. One way of doing this is to add calories to what they would normally eat and drink. If your dad normally eats porridge made with salt and water, add some cream to the recipe.

If the person you are trying to support is older and frail, they may have a smaller appetite and eat sparingly, which means you have to get all the calories and vitamins they need into smaller amounts of food. Nearly everyone knows the difference between fattening and non-fattening foods these days. For a person who does not eat much, the richer the food the better. They still need the fibre that comes from vegetables, but you can dress them with rich sauces, or butter, to keep the calories high.

When we have mashed potatoes I make them with cream and butter. My mother eats like a bird, but I can tempt her with little pots of full-fat yoghurt and as many chocolate gingers as she wants. (Daughter living at home with her mother)

Difficulty in swallowing can affect people with dementia. This can be associated with a loss of coordination skills. It might help if you think about the mechanics of chewing and swallowing. First the food has to get into your mouth, and eyesight or difficulties with cutlery can be a problem. Then you have to manipulate it into a soft ball of food that can be swallowed, and this requires saliva, which may be reduced in old age and with some medicines or dehydration. Sore gums and mouth ulcers or poor teeth can be a problem, so you need to get the dentist to take a look. The tongue then coordinates pushing the food back into the throat without allowing it to go into the lungs, thus causing choking. A speech therapist can advise on what sort of consistency of food is best at various stages of dementia. To begin with, keep going with everything that is popular. In the end, perhaps some items need to be softened. Curiously, mixed textures in one mouthful are sometimes a problem, like soup with bits, or crunchy cereal in milk.

The perfect meal

A great meal is when everyone is relaxed and happy, with the food that is served to your taste and in exactly the right amounts. You've got enough time to eat it and, if you have company, enough time to socialise over it, and you are not worrying about how it is going to be paid for. The surroundings are comfortable and you are not distracted by noise or harassed by the people serving the meal. Any faux pas like dropping your cutlery, or having to spit out an unexpected bone or olive stone, can be overcome discreetly, and any spills or drips are dealt with using your lovely big napkin. Many care homes achieve this with people who are very disabled by their dementia, but some do not, and hospitals have been notoriously unfocused on this issue. You may need to keep an eye on this for your loved one even while they are at home. And if the person can't sit still for all that, finger food and snacking are great ways to get enough calories in, washed down by frequent hot and cold drinks, available on demand. *Bon appetit!*

Keeping a calm environment

Having dementia is very worrying. The stress leads to upsetting behaviour, and people find that hard to deal with at home. Many of the inconvenient problems of dementia can be worked out using some of the ideas in this book, but all of them will be solved more easily if there is a relaxed atmosphere. If someone is shouting, repeating themselves, refusing to eat, trying to go out in unsuitable clothes (sometimes all at the same time!), staying cool and tranquil would be a miracle. So the secret is to put as much in place as possible to keep a stress-free background environment. This means avoiding over-stimulation – and everyone has different things that they find stimulating, so you have to decide for yourself what will work in your situation. Also remember that stress is contagious. A relaxed carer feeling good will help the person with dementia.

Here are some hints for keeping a calm environment in the house:

- Exercise reduces stress and burns off excess energy that could give rise to difficult behaviour. Taking someone with dementia for a nice long walk often reduces the chaos in the home that is created by endless attempts to stop them disappearing out the front or the back door and getting lost. The person with dementia, even after they have started to get lost at times, can go for walks on their own, if you have a suitable tracking device. Friends who are looking for a role might help with this. A dog is a good companion for this sort of work.

- Talking of dogs ... research shows that petting an animal can reduce your blood pressure and caring for it gives many health benefits. Even if the person with dementia does not speak any more, they can still communicate and the dog knows it is loved, and will come back again and again for scratches and pats. A recent development has been the 'dementia dog', which is a trained companion animal for people with dementia. It can do a variety of clever tasks, like remind you to take your pills. But a major benefit arises from the fact that the general public is sentimental about working dogs. The dementia dog with his smart working coat invites interaction with other people who want to pat the dog, and his job is a good subject for conversation when the dog is out walking with his master or mistress. The responsibility and routine of caring for the dog add to the motivation for the owner. (Dogs get dementia too, but that is another story ...)

As the handler put the cat into the bed, the patient suddenly awoke, removed his arms from under the sheets and started to pet the cat. I truly believe animals have special healing powers and a sixth sense ... Edward Creagan of the Mayo Clinic Medical School observed, 'If pet ownership was a medication, it would be patented tomorrow.' (Sherri Snelling, founder of the CareGiver Club)

- If you haven't got a dog to cuddle, you are just going to have to cuddle each other. Touch is very important. If you are a family that never had much body contact, now is a good time to start. Have big hugs and learn the pleasure of sitting on the sofa beside your mum, stroking her hair or rubbing some nice cream into her feet and ankles. Get her to do that for you. You need care as well. You could go on a course and learn massage, but gentle stroking does not need theory – just practice. And consider getting a massage for yourself. If you've not tried it you are really missing out.

- Keep the stimulation level right. This might mean keeping the noise down, as recommended for communication in Chapter 9. It might mean making sure the hearing aids are working so that the person is not frustrated by not being able to hear. There can be too much noise and too little noise and you will know what is best at each time of the day. Try sitting quietly on your own with your eyes shut and just listen to the house ... there may be noises of which you were not aware. It is often the case at night, when the person with dementia being disturbing is particularly inconvenient. Gentle music (preferred music, chosen by the person with dementia) can drown out other extraneous noises. Radio programmes with their attention-grabbing breaks in the music and jingles might be disturbing. But then, if your person with dementia is a heavy metal fan, you'll possibly set them off by playing quiet background music. Only you can tell, but make sure that you are aware of the situation and use all the knowledge you have about what matters most to the person with dementia.

- There are commercial companies selling packages for retailers which combine music and scent that they claim will reduce perceived waiting time in shops and make us spend more money in hotels and restaurants. People in marketing departments know that smells can make a difference to our behaviour. We know this from the effect on us of the smell of bread in the supermarket (which perhaps comes from a canister and not an oven). Domestic versions of the scent idea are available which release pulsed whiffs of smells that are likely to improve the atmosphere. It's not just about covering bad odours with a burst of so-called 'fragrance of the forest'. For example, the smell of Bakewell tart is scientifically proven to increase appetite. A well-fed person is more content and calm, and maybe one of those scent machines could help with the ideas of pages 129–130 for stimulating a failing appetite.

According to psychologist Maria Larsson, 'The two cerebral structures, the amygdala and the hippocampus, play an important role for the storing of memories, and the olfactory nerve has very direct connections to both structures.'

Help your family member with dementia feel the strong emotions and warm memories associated with smells by popping a batch of cookies in the oven, go for a walk just after it rains, fold the laundry together, or come up with activity ideas of your own that will generate aromas particularly significant to your loved one. Sawdust, a campfire, garlic bread, a fine red wine, perfume, pine, and soap are just a few ideas of scents that may unlock rich, emotional memories and bring comfort to someone with dementia. (Quoted in www. helpforalzheimersfamilies.com)

However, the discussion posts on the Help for Alzheimer's Families website show that there can be problems with sensory loss.

My husband has lost his sense of smell and taste. He chews tobacco (nastily, I might add) and has false teeth. It becomes so hard to deal with him …

Design ideas

The key design ideas are covered in Chapter 9, but it is worth summarising the basics here:

- In a familiar environment change as little as possible.
- In a new environment make everything as plain and obvious as possible, including signage when needed.
- In both cases increasing the light level can make more difference than the medication for some people.
- Use all the assistive technology that is available to you, and start using it at the earliest possible stage. This will maximise the opportunity for the person with dementia to become familiar with it and for you to learn how to maintain and use it.

Activity ideas

There is a roaring trade within the dementia field in courses and books on activities for people with dementia. In truth, if you want to stay at home for as long as possible the important thing is to keep busy. This means doing everything you usually do, whether that's bowling, gardening, going to church, visiting museums or simply getting out and about to the shops. Anything that involves exercise, socialising and mental stimulation should be at the top of your list. Festering in front of the television is probably not on that list, but everyone has their moments when they need to do that – just as long as it doesn't stop you going out and talking to people. Pretend you are having a little nap, because naps are good for people with dementia. And the TV is so boring, you might actually doze off. Remember to put your feet up and get comfy.

Disturbing behaviour

There is more about how to manage 'disturbing behaviour' in Chapter 8. However, because people with dementia can make life difficult for those they live with or for their neighbours, it can lead to them having to lose their home. Sometimes this is because they've got a problem that they can't communicate using language like they used to, so they behave in upsetting ways until the underlying problem is solved. You know this person very well, so you can create your own checklist of what may be causing the problem.

- Is the light bright enough?
- Do they need the toilet?
- Are they in pain?
- Is hunger or thirst the problem?
- Do they need to get out and about?
- Is the room too hot or too cold?
- Is there some noise or other disturbance that they can't understand and don't like?
- Are other people in the environment being annoying?
- Is there a medication problem?

If you are doing everything recommended in this book to try to keep the situation calm and happy but it is not working you need to get advice. Some people involved with dementia don't like the use of the term 'disturbing behaviour' and this is explored in Chapter 8.

There are certain behaviours that people find particularly difficult. Sexual disinhibition, not dressing properly and being verbally inappropriate are hard to manage. Incontinence presents real practical problems if it seems that the person is deliberately urinating or opening their bowels in the wrong place. Look for help in Chapter 8.

Security

People with dementia often maintain a good daily routine in the familiarity of their own home, but family and friends worry about them and excessive caution can lead to a premature move into care. When you live a long way from your relative, being actively involved in their care can be frightening if you don't have much idea of what they are up to.

Mum's neighbour has my number in Kansas and he called to say that she'd been seen in her garden in her nightclothes at five in the morning. I didn't know what to do. I called her and she had no idea what I was talking about. (Ken, son of Agnes, 72)

Family carers can exhaust themselves trying to visit frequently to check on the person and the visits might be impossible if you are in Kansas. Even if you are local a quick check round the door is of little value to the person with dementia, as there is not time enough to do much. There is an electronic system called 'Just Checking' that provides families with a daily activity / movement chart that can be followed online. It is used by social services in some areas to work out what support the person needs most and when. Small wireless sensors placed around the house are triggered in the main rooms when the person moves around. That data is automatically recorded and can be viewed at any time by the family logging into the checking-system website using a password. It is not a web camera, so it is very private. The sort of thing they can see is whether the person got in and out of bed a lot during the night, or had unexpected visitors or care calls. You can see if the person left the house, and the system can generate an alert to you if the person leaves the house at an unexpected time, such as five in the morning.

The council installed a checking system, and we'll never know what it was that got her out on the street on those two occasions that the neighbour saw her because she's never done it since. I even wonder if she did it before ... that neighbour's a bit strange himself. I wonder if he wanted me to get her out of there and into a home for some other reason. He's always wanted to buy her house. (Ken, son of Agnes, 72)

There is more about practical ways of managing what is often called 'wandering' in Chapter 8. Some people don't like the use of that expression because it implies that the moving about is senseless, when in fact the problem is that we have not tried hard enough to make sense of it.

Other security issues arise when the person with dementia is worried about too many of their door keys circulating in the community. A biometric lock that is operated by fingerprints can help, or the more traditional key safe, which is a secure box attached to the outside of the house containing a spare house key. The person on the outside accesses the key safe using a secret code, and uses the key to open the door before returning it to the box for the next visitor. You can see more equipment like this on the ATDementia website (see Resources and helpful organisations, page 320).

Rest, respite and home care

Health and social care services and voluntary organisations often offer day care services that will help to maintain someone at home. The private sector also has a long tradition of offering these services. If money is no object you can have all of them, but even if you are reliant on health and social care, many of them may be available if they assess you as needing them and they have the resources.

- Complex care services can be provided at home when someone has been discharged from hospital and has significant nursing care needs that require continuous monitoring.

- Night care is available where the agency provides a nurse, carer or support worker to support sleeping and to deal with any disturbances or care needs in the night. They can help with bathing and getting someone ready for bed, and they will provide drinks. They can even wear night-time clothes to help avoid confusion when the person wakes up. The night-time person can arrange to be awake all the time, or retire to sleep and be on call when you need them.

- When the person with dementia approaches the end of life, there is a great temptation from NHS services to transfer them to hospital even though health care professionals could provide care round the clock at home. We are familiar with Macmillan nurses undertaking this for people with cancer, but people at the end of life with other diagnoses such as dementia can also be helped by twenty-four-hour care.

- Holiday care can be provided in the person's own home so that the carer can go away. Some agencies will even offer a hotel call out service, so that you could get help at your holiday location if you go away together.

- Live-in care is available from agencies for varying lengths of time, not just holiday respite.

- Hospital to home services can support a person who wants to go back home after a hospital admission.

- Help with household activities, the daily routine, day trips out and social activities can be what enables someone to stay at home. Families can do a lot, but in their absence voluntary organisations and other friends can be invaluable.

It's important to remember that the majority of people with dementia stay at home in the last weeks of their lives, and this is achievable, even if it takes a bit of organising. There is a high likelihood that any one of us will have difficulty in arranging to die in our own bed at home. Many people get rushed to hospital at the end – at times without any real benefit. Advance directives and other mechanisms described in Chapter 13 will give you some idea of how to avoid that, if you want to think about it at all.

Chapter 8

Disturbing behaviours

Most of the time, things will be just as they always were. You are living with the same person. However, the dementia will at some stage make the person you know behave in new ways that cause you and them stress and distress. This chapter will help you with ideas for avoiding that sort of disturbing behaviour and suggest ways of dealing with it together. People with dementia say they get irritated when they are treated in a different way by those they live with, above all in the early stages of their condition, so remember that your husband, wife, parent or other loved one is still the person they were yesterday.

When we came out of the clinic and they'd told me it was dementia I was in shock. It was an even bigger shock when I realised the wife wouldn't even let me take the rubbish out in case I got lost. (Don, 73)

Sadly, later in the journey people with dementia do eventually present problems from time to time, both to themselves and to their families when they are living together, because of disturbing behaviour. You will not experience all of these tribulations, and if they do happen they are unlikely to be a permanent characteristic. As dementia progresses, symptoms come and go. Research has shown that there are six areas that present the greatest test for carers. These are:

- aggression;
- agitation or anxiety;
- depression;
- hallucinations and delusions;
- sleeplessness;
- wandering.

Medication has only a limited role in dealing with any of these. If the person is on dementia-specific medication, it helps. The other medications that doctors might prescribe include sedatives that may not work and can have bad side effects. Others, like non-sedative antidepressants, can be useful in anxiety and depression, but the fewer drugs one has to take the better. In this chapter I am going to suggest non-drug responses to each of these six challenges based on the original advice in the booklet *10 Helpful Hints for Carers*. These are strategies that you can try on your own at home that we know from research or experience can make a difference. Of course, you may try all of them and find they don't work. At that stage you really need professional help.

Aggression

An important note is that if your relationship is with someone who was always violent, this is a different and difficult case and you need to ask for help at once. Start with your GP. Frontotemporal dementia, the one that affects the front of the brain, can give rise to aggression, because the frontal lobes of the brain are the place where your inhibitions lie. The psychiatric team or the GP can tell you about this in advance so that you can anticipate problems and let the team know if and when they become an issue. In other sorts of dementia it can occur simply because of what is going on. Aggression does not occur in every person with dementia, and generally that is only for a short time, but it is always shocking, because it is most likely to hurt those who are trying to help. You can approach this problem in a number of ways.

- Leave the room. It is imperative to keep yourself out of harm's way. Giving the person time and space to calm down is helpful. You remove any possible annoyance that you personally have innocently caused and it means that you are safer. The proverb says 'Sticks and stones will break my bones, names will never hurt me', but this is not strictly true. Even verbal aggression will affect your well-being, so give yourself a break. Walking away also removes you from the understandable but completely unacceptable temptation to hit back. It gives both parties time and space to calm down, and allows you time to work out who you can turn to. It is not your fault but the result of the condition, and do not be afraid to ask for help, even if you think what is happening is shameful.

I woke up and found my husband beside the bed brandishing a knife. He said, 'What have you done with my wife, you evil bitch. I don't know who you are, but you better get out of here!' (Edith, 79)

- It is really very tough, but do everything in your power not to argue with a person who has dementia. There is no point and it will create an atmosphere that will make things worse. Even if you manage to convince them that the thought they have is wrong, they may forget that position very soon and start back on the old tack. The problem is that people get a sort of emotional hangover, where they feel angry and suspicious long after the occurrence that caused those feelings. Try to avoid 'No, but …' and replace it with 'Yes, and …' If you don't you may inadvertently create more trouble for yourself.

Mr Smith was a gentle and devoted husband with one hobby, betting on the horses on a Saturday. His wife had always kept the family finances, so he asked her for a tenner for his bet once a week. When dementia set in he started asking for the money randomly, and more than once a day. If she argued that he'd had it, or it was not Saturday, he got really angry and rough with her. She could not give him money every time he asked because he frequently hid it, lost it or gave it away, and it could be up to £50 or £60 a day. The son came up with a great solution: persuading his mother not to argue but to hand out a reproduction old-style ten-pound note (badly copied to avoid fear of forgery accusations, the sort that is used as a stage prop) every time Mr Smith asked. The only people who complained were the grandchildren, who sometimes got given them as pocket money. He never actually did go out to the bookies. He just needed to know he could whenever he wanted, because to him it is always Saturday. (Dementia nurse)

- Check if the person is in pain. Undiagnosed and untreated pain is one of the common causes of disturbing behaviour in dementia. Even if they are not complaining of pain it might be at the root of the behaviour. Your doctor can help with this. If taking tablets is an issue, consider transdermal patches – pain patches that are put on like a sticking plaster and deliver slow-release analgesia through the skin.

- Work out if there are any noticeable triggers for the disturbing behaviour. Aggression is a coherent response from a person who misinterprets what is happening because of deficits in their understanding and recall. They know something is wrong and they are angry and scared, so they fight. If you see the world from their point of view, you'll understand why it actually makes sense to fight. If they've always been confident and competent and everything seems to be going wrong, they might do something extreme. As the person tries to work out where they are and what is going on, they make mistakes. Is this a bathroom or a storeroom? Is the person trying to undress them a nurse or a rapist? The violent resistance to being cared for is logical within the world view of a person who cannot remember or work things out and may be experiencing hallucinations. There are design ideas in Chapter 9 that might help with this. Keep a diary about the person's moods and get a sense of what sets them off and what they find relaxing and comforting. You are going to have to talk to professionals about this, and details of what happens and when will help them decide how they can help you and assess the level of risk that you have.

My mother suddenly decided she disliked baths and my dad was able to muddle through until she had a bad fall. When she came back from hospital for a while nurses came in to help with washing – it was a disaster. Mum got aggressive and called the Nigerian nurse a 'darkie', much to my dad's shame. I can understand that you don't want strangers manhandling you, but basic hygiene is important. We're still wrestling with this one. (Ruth, whose mother has dementia)

Experienced professionals and care workers must never put up with racial abuse, but in practice are able to distinguish when it is the illness talking and respond with forbearance and dignity.

● Think of taking them walking and offer as much opportunity for exercise as possible. Fresh air and exercise can help with mood and natural fatigue reduces stress. You might be starting to wonder if I believe that exercise solves everything, but to be honest it has amazing value. The person with dementia will find it harder to fight if they are tired. Although some people get irritable when tired, it's possible that a long walk will make them more likely to nap than snap.

- Try to avoid future outbursts by creating a calm environment. There is advice on this in Chapter 7. How you do it will be different for every individual. Find out what works and keep doing it.

- Make life less challenging. When a person starts to forget how to use everyday objects the frustration is maddening. People with dementia sometimes become disinhibited, and where once they would have gritted their teeth, they may now just lose their self-control. Fear leads to violence.

- Touch and comforting words that work when the person is anxious may also work to ward off aggression, but make sure that the touch is not misunderstood as restraint, because the person will attempt to get away, perhaps hurting you and themselves in the process.

Agitation or anxiety

Agitation in a person with dementia can be generated by a range of issues, so you have to be a detective and find out what usually causes it in this person in order to avoid those triggers. What's bothering a person with dementia gets amplified because they've lost the capacity to distract themselves or to move away from what is upsetting. Their behaviour may be restless or clingy, and they may cry out.

- Protect yourself from the strain that arises when you are living with an agitated person. If they are inconsolable for long periods it will give rise to strong feelings in you, such as anger, frustration or resentfulness. You might start to feel hopeless about the situation. You need to take breaks away and to keep up your own emotional, social and spiritual supports as much as you can.

- See if there is an underlying physical problem. Does the agitated person have pain or an unmet need, such as hunger or thirst? You might take them to the doctor to see if there is any undiagnosed clinical condition.

- Touching and holding can really help, as long as the person does not think you are trying to restrain them. In agitation the person has an overwhelming feeling that they need to get away and their body is flooded with the hormones for 'flight or fight', so if you restrain them you are restricting their choice and all that's left is 'fight'. This is best avoided. If you have never tried massage, now is the time. The combination of a peaceful setting, restful music, perhaps candlelight and scented oils, and the comfort from the physical touch to loosen knotted muscles can really help. If you are not up to that, just rubbing someone's hands or feet with cream or stroking their hair may help, if they will let you.

- The agitated person might pace about and so you can use up some of this energy with purposeful exercise.

  Dad used to get in a right state cooped up in the house. I'd get him out in the garden and ask him to help me dig the potato patch. We never put any potatoes in there, but it got a good digging over and he seemed more relaxed after. (Son, speaking about his retired father, who had been a refuse collector)

- Aromatherapy has been the subject of serious research in dementia. No one quite knows why it works. The person with dementia, particularly if they are very old, has a reduced sense of smell, so researchers think it's not necessarily the nice smell that makes it work. Lemon balm and lavender have produced significant reductions in agitated behaviour, including sleeplessness and wandering. It seems not only to be the personal attention or massage that makes the difference, because essential oils work better than vegetable oil. It has been wondered if the reduced agitation is as a result of the calming effect on the carer of administering this nice treatment. Worth a try, but make sure that you follow the instructions for use of essential oils.

● A calming atmosphere can help a lot. It is most soothing for a person at home if as little as possible is changed. You may make some small changes so that the place is safer under foot, in order to avoid falls that could lead to a hospital admission. There is more about creating a calm atmosphere in Chapter 7.

● Because the person does not remember the passage of time, they may start to look for lost possessions. You might agree one day to replace an old chair and then the person starts to look for it again the following day and wonder what's happened to it. We all forget things like this from time to time, but in dementia because it happens so often the person might be made agitated by the constant sense that something is changing without their control.

I'm sure the toilet used to be here. (Jack, 85, pointing to the cupboard under the stairs)

It's important not to add to the anxiety by arguing, but distraction can make a difference. Jack's daughter can say, 'Well, here it is now, behind this other door.' And putting a clear label on the toilet door or leaving the door open for the toilet to be seen is a good way of distracting the person from looking for it fruitlessly in the wrong place.

● People who have agitation sometimes seem to benefit from light therapy or daylight lamps. These are meant to have the same effect as being outside in daylight, because they give off the same spectrum of light. Walking in the open air would be even better, but sometimes this is not practical. Keep the house as full of light as possible, using the design ideas listed in Chapter 9. Daylight lamps are also said to help with depression.

● Music is such good medicine it should be available on the NHS. However, just as you need to take the right medicine, so it needs to be the right music. In order to make the correct choice you need to know a lot about the person. Research shows that music still has meaning and a positive effect for a person with dementia and their carer up to the very end of life.

● There is a movement in dementia care which is called 'Life Story Work'. This means working with the person to find out interesting and important things about their life. What you consider most fascinating may not be what they regard as important to them. For example, you might think that it was most significant that someone was a great army general, but his most memorable experience might be that he wrote and published a children's book. Of course everything from someone's past defines them to an extent, but it's important to go beyond the obvious things that everyone knows about a person and get close to what matters to them. There may be topics they wish to avoid, because they find them painful. On the other hand, people do sometimes find comfort in thinking about the past even if it was sad, and shedding a tear, before going on to think of something else. In general, though, it's meant to be fun. Creating a scrapbook is a practical way of working on this, and you end up with something that other people can use to stimulate conversation, or to sit and quietly look through as a distraction when the person is agitated. If you are able to create a digital version of the scrapbook and print it out or share it on a laptop or other device, this will guard against the risk of the material getting lost or destroyed. You can also share that version with relatives all over the world to find out if they have any more reminiscences or ideas or photos to add to the story. There are templates for such books in the references at the end of the book.

Depression

● Activities that relieve boredom or provide distraction can help with depression. Anyone who is bored or inactive may feel down and fed up. You know this person well, so you know what would cheer them up.

When Mum gets down I stick her in the car and take her down to the shopping centre and we sit in the food hall watching the world go by. Then we go round the shoe shops and shock ourselves with the price of shoes and the terrible high heels that girls wear these days. (Son, 60)

● A dog or cat is a great companion for people who need cheering up. It does not matter how depressed his owner is, the dog still needs a walk. Fresh air, exercise and daylight will help to combat those low feelings and also be good for the dog. Cats provide companionship in a less demanding way and are easier to keep.

● Remembering the past is a great distraction from depression. When people are losing some of their capacity, you need to be aware that much of the stuff they know from the past will be lost if you don't ask them about it now. Our oral tradition of telling stories is not just about the preservation of the stories but also about the great pleasure of telling them and listening to them, even when they are familiar.

Tell me again, Granny, about when you jumped on top of the wedding cake because they would not let you be a bridesmaid. (A.B., 11)

You need to learn the trick of starting a really good conversation about the past, and take the person out of their gloomy spiral of thoughts.

● There is research that suggests you can make things better using 'multisensory therapy', which involves stimulating the person with music and light, and even nice smells, to lift them from their depression. You can buy a machine with fibre-optic strands to play with and lights that change their colour. In some care homes they have whole rooms with this equipment. It is often not used, so if there is one, try it out when you are visiting. Because it is hardly ever used, I'd hesitate to install one, but if it is there, have a look.

● Although it's wrong to argue, there is a great temptation when someone is depressed to try to correct them about what is getting them down.

The old lady was crying because she'd been told her mother was dead. She cried as if her mother had died yesterday. Her mum died fifty years ago. I heard her husband going on and on at her to remind her that they all went to the funeral before their children were even born. (Dementia nurse)

There is an alternative way of dealing with this raw emotion called 'validation'. Instead of making her out to be wrong, because it would be frightening and depressing to be made to understand that she is losing her grip on reality on top of the utter sense of bereavement, the best response is to go with the flow of the feelings – which are 'valid' under the circumstances.

I advised him not to tell her again that her mother was long dead. He thought she should know and she'd get over it if she was reminded that it was long ago. Instead I took her on to the sofa and put my arms round her and said, 'Oh, your mother is a lovely lady, isn't she? Is she a good cook? Tell me all about what she's like …' I drifted into the past tense. 'Did she use bones for soup or a stock cube?' (Dementia nurse)

It does not really matter whether she is wrong about when her mother died. The important thing is to offer comfort, because it is right to feel grief. Most of us feel less pain over time after someone has died. We still love them and their memory, but it does not hurt so much. If you have forgotten that the time has passed, your grief feels very new and genuine and should be treated as such. You can't be argued out of it. The solution is gentle distraction. It must be a nightmare to live through these storms of emotion.

When I was training to be a nurse forty years ago I was asked to wake a man who had alcohol-related brain damage. He was a heavy drinker anyway, but his wife died in a car crash and he drank himself into oblivion. When I went to his room he seemed bewildered. 'Where am I?' 'In hospital.' He swore loud and long and cheerfully. 'What happened? What time is it?' I started to try to tell him that he needed to come for breakfast, but he started grabbing his clothes and shoes to dress quickly. 'She'll be waiting for me off the night shift. Oh, my God, I'll be in trouble.' In a quiet firm voice I told him his wife was dead, he was ill, and he needed to come for breakfast. He would not believe me at first, but when he looked in my face and I repeated it he crumpled up and sobbed. I confessed later to the charge nurse that I felt I had not handled it well, and should have treated it more like breaking bad news than correcting his confusion. 'Never mind,' he sighed. 'I'll give you another shot with him tomorrow morning when he wakes, and each day for the rest of the week.' (Retired psychiatric nurse)

Comfort and distraction is what is needed, not logical argument. Apart from anything else, you may have to go through this a number of times. You need to make it easy on yourself. Don't argue about anything. Nothing will be gained on either side, neither insight nor satisfaction.

- Many dementia organisations recommend counselling as a help for depression. The research that has been done so far does not suggest that it makes a great difference, but when you see how often it is recommended by those who should know, it must be worth trying. The counsellor needs to know that the client has dementia as some of the commonly used techniques don't work for people with dementia.

- Companionship of other people is hugely important. People with dementia, particularly in the early stages, get a huge amount of support from joining a group of people like themselves. Contact your local Alzheimer's organisation to find out where there is one or ask the community psychiatric nurse if they are going to start one. Dementia support groups are a great place to talk in safety about subjects that are of concern. Not least, they are a place of great happiness.

I am a professor in the field and I take it all very seriously. The people in the dementia working group, all of whom have dementia, have me rocking with laughter. It is about dementia, about themselves, about how others treat them. Of course they are angry and sad, but they share their laughter generously and tell me it is better than any medicine. (June Andrews, in 10 Helpful Hints for Carers)

- As with the person who faces aggression or agitation, the person living with someone who has depression needs to care for themselves as well in order not to be dragged down by the circumstances. If the person you are looking after is beyond consolation, you need to contact someone and your GP will be the first port of call. Sometimes people with dementia (and their carers) can develop a clinical depressive illness that is more than an ordinary response to the stress of the situation. You need support, which might include medication.

Hallucinations and delusions

A hallucination is the experience of seeing or hearing something that is not there. In fact you can hallucinate with any of your five senses. It's different from an illusion. I might think I see a face in the pattern on the carpet, but when I concentrate I can see it is only a carpet. That would be an illusion. A hallucination would be when I see a face in the carpet and even if the pattern or shadow is pointed out to me I still believe there is someone there and won't accept that I am mistaken. It's more common in Lewy body dementia than in other forms. The brain is constantly trying to make sense of the messages it receives and if it is not working properly it 'invents' something to make sense of the poorly processed information it has.

My dad is tortured with the Lewy body. At night, he'll be shouting and swearing and fighting with enemies that aren't there. He can see them and hear them. And mother is trying to sleep down the stairs because she's afraid he'll hit her. He doesn't mean it. And in the morning he apologises. Always. It's almost worse that he realises what he's been like. It's a living nightmare. (Son of Mr B., who has Parkinson's disease and Lewy body dementia)

A delusion is a fixed false belief that is contrary to culture and implausible. You might think that your dad already has a number of fixed false beliefs: for example, that his football team might win the league, or that we don't notice his bald patch under the comb-over – these are reasonable bits of self-delusion shared by many men in our culture. Don't go there, because his ideas are almost plausible. However, if he believes that someone is stealing from him or that your mum is having an affair when clearly she is a frail little grandmother who has only ever loved one man, this is a delusion. It's not credible. It is the result of the disease and you have to decide what to do about it to look after them both. The general rules are about distraction, making sure the person is well and avoiding arguments.

It may be that he has forgotten that he disposed of something and is now looking for it and assumes that it must have been stolen. He may be having difficulty remembering how long his wife has been out of the house on an errand and putting two and two together to make five about her behaviour. There may be something in the past that is surfacing for him. There is no point in trying to get to the bottom of any of that. The most important thing is to stop anyone getting upset, if it can be avoided.

The issue about culture is important in deciding what is a delusion. A person with dementia might be said to be deluded because they believe an angel is by their side all day that no one can see. Before deciding to act upon this, remember that not all delusions are frightening and bad, and this might not even be a delusion for all you know. You might decide to leave a source of comfort as it is.

One really difficult situation is when the person has a fixed, false belief that they need to go home for some reason. The wail of distress when you tell a mother that she can't go home to her child is real, even if the child is long grown up and gone away. That sort of feeling is a kind of delusion and the most effective response again is distraction.

The general rules of thumb for hallucinations and delusions are similar.

- It is a good idea not to argue with a person who has dementia, ever. Arguing about the existence of the object that is being hallucinated, or the voices or smell or sound, is fruitless. Another way of saying this is that you should not try to 'prove' anything. If your mother hallucinates and thinks small animals surround her chair she'll be distressed if you trample all over the carpet to prove they are not there. She'll be as distressed as she would be if they were real. Her distress will continue long after she's forgotten what you did to upset her. You won't be able to argue your father out of the idea of thieves or infidelity. You can only distract him from his anger and get him out of her way till he forgets it.

So when he started on about her having an affair, I just said, 'Good grief. Have you seen the time? We were supposed to be at the town centre half an hour ago to pick up my nephew.' And I got him into his coat and into the car and we went to a café, and when the nephew did not turn up (which would have been a miracle, because he lives in London now) we had a pot of tea and went home. (Son of Mr B.)

You may have to repeat the exercise. Some delusions stick around for a bit.

- If you increase the light level and make everything clear, you can at least reduce the likelihood that the person with dementia is also struggling with illusions.

Another bad day today. I saw my reflection in the lounge plate-glass window after dark and started yelling at Moira that the neighbours were in our garden and that she should call the police. Of course, it turned out to be me. (Gerald, 68)

As illusions may arise from confusion caused by mirrors, and reflections, covering up windows with nets or closing curtains at night helps. A bright light in the garden at night that might prevent the mirror-like reflections back into the room from windows is another possible strategy.

● Fortunately, hallucinations in dementia are not always unpleasant. This is in marked contrast to the hallucinations suffered by people with depression. However, if the image was horrible and frightening, it is better to give comfort than try to persuade them that their anxiety was unfounded. It has been suggested that the person is more likely to hallucinate if there is not much going on. It appears that some people with dementia hallucinate and are aware of the hallucination but are able to 'tune out' of it. It has been said it's like having the TV on but not watching it; or like having someone talking in the room to whom you are paying no attention. They are still aware of it but they screen it out, which is harder to do if there is nothing much else happening.

● Avoid boredom for the same reason. However, it is important to note that stress makes hallucinations more likely. It's tricky. If you over-stimulate or under-stimulate you add to the problem. Knowing the person really well will help you to judge it right. The symptoms more frequently strike in the evening. The person may be conscious or drowsy and inaccessible. Hallucinations are usually visual, but a small number of people experience sounds or voices that are not there and some experience smells.

Well, you ask me about distraction? To be honest, it's whatever works. One of my patients can be distracted over and over by the same DVD on the television. Others will refuse to enjoy their usual entertainment when they are disturbed and so a walk outside works best – just to tire them out a bit. Remember that most of us can be distracted by words, or conversation, but the person with dementia may be getting less

*verbal and more non-verbal. It's whatever works for that individual.
The really clever thing is if you can work out what it is that sets them
off, and do something about that. (Dementia adviser)*

● You have to make sure that the person has enough to eat and
drink and enough sleep.

● You can ask the pharmacist or doctor to review the medication,
because some combinations can cause a problem. On the other
hand, it might be another physical illness (that can be treated)
that is making the situation worse. The doctor may be able to
offer medication that might make a difference. There are risks
if antipsychotic medication is used, but it can help some people.
It might even be that an eye and hearing test would help to
prevent the sorts of illusions or misperceptions that precede
hallucinations or precipitate delusions.

*Mary was sure that the neighbours were prowling round her garden at
night and she got quite paranoid about it, but the situation improved
radically after we'd got her hearing aids and her glasses fixed.
(Daughter of Mary, 75)*

● If the hallucinations are not scary and they are not getting in
the way of daily living, you might not worry about them too
much, as long as you've checked with the doctor that there is
nothing preventable. Understanding the cause should make
you less worried, but make sure you've asked to see if there is
anything that can be fixed.

● Remember the squirrel.

*My mum kept saying to me when I asked her how she was, 'Oh,
don't worry about me. Basil keeps me company. He comes round for
afternoon tea.' We assumed that she had an imaginary friend because
we knew about the hallucinations and delusions and she'd had*

Parkinson's. I wondered if we should tell the doctor. The children even joined in talking about Basil. When I was doing her blinds one day I saw this squirrel on the washing pole and when I pointed it out to her she said, 'Of course, that's old Basil. Open the window and he'll come in for his treats.' (From 10 Helpful Hints for Carers)

This daughter assumed that there was a hallucination or a delusion when there was neither.

Sleeplessness

When people talk about the stress of caring and the physical illnesses that carers suffer, a lot is down to inadequate sleep. It is hard to rest when you have to keep one eye open all night because someone in the house has developed nocturnal behaviours. Sleep deprivation is used as torture, and we all know why.

- Here we go again with the exercise advice! If people get exercise they sleep better. It is possible to exercise in the house, with chair exercises and dancing and moving about. But exercise that exposes you to daylight, particularly in the early part of the day, is especially good for you. The reason is explained in Chapter 9 in the section on light (see page 176).

- At every stage of life having a bedtime routine is important for getting people to settle. You know what works best in your house. However, it is worth noting the obvious things. Screen time should be stopped an hour or two before settling, because the light stimulation does affect the body clock. Whatever is comforting, like a milky drink or a warm bath, provide these things if you can – make them part of a familiar routine. Everyone should know that when the telly goes off and the cocoa is poured out it is nearly time to turn in.

● Even in care homes now, night staff are being issued with dressing gowns so that if someone wakes up in the night they are not met with the spectacle of people walking about in daytime clothes. They will then get the impression that they are disturbing other sleepers and are more receptive to being encouraged back into bed. Putting away daytime objects like clothes and shoes gives visual cues to the fact that it is bedtime.

It's logical to me. I was a nurse all my working life. If I end up in a care home and wake up in the night and see lots of staff milling about in uniform, I'll probably get up and ask for jobs to do. If our residents get up and see us in the dressing gowns it is easier to put your finger to your lips and say, 'Shhh! Don't wake everyone up. Let's go back to your room and I'll bring you a nice cup of tea so you can settle down till morning ...' (Jane, care manager)

● People sleep better in a cool room with a warm bed. Just being too hot can make the person inclined to get up for a wander. If they then see that the outside light is on they may go out to investigate. Better to encourage a quick trip to the loo before snuggling down again by keeping the room cooler.

When my mother went for respite to the care home the staff made a big issue about her not sleeping but wandering about and they got the doctor to prescribe sleeping pills for it. I was very annoyed and pointed out that the radiator in her room could not be turned down and she was uncomfortable with the unaccustomed heat at night. They said there was nothing that could be done, but I complained to the manager and a heating engineer repaired the control on her radiator that day. It was nonsense. (Hazel, daughter of M., 85)

● Talking of light, it is important to keep the room as dark as possible, particularly if this is what the person is used to, or if they are accustomed to a small night-light. Darkness has a physiological effect on the body. In Scotland, in summer, the daylight creeps in at 4.30 a.m. – a time to get some blackout blinds. Even moonlight interferes with sleepiness.

● The most common reason for getting out of bed at night is to go to the toilet. If you have an en suite toilet and you can position the bed so that the toilet can be seen when the person's head is on the pillow, that is an ideal arrangement. When using the toilet they can see the comfy bed and when in bed they can see the toilet. The greatest problem is when the person starts to wander round the house looking for, and even forgetting that they are looking for, the toilet and then being unable to find their way back to bed.

● By the time we are old, most of us have developed a variety of aches and pains. Taking a painkiller half an hour before bedtime might mean that those creaky joints and tired muscles don't get in the way of dropping off to sleep. Talk to the doctor about whether over-the-counter medicines are advisable and if they will be enough. We all know the danger of mixing drugs and alcohol, and so it is worth having a chat with the doctor about this while you are there. A small alcoholic drink might help the person to drop off. Too much is counterproductive, as anyone who drinks a lot may be wakeful in the early hours when the effects start to wear off. Ask the doctor if a glass of stout or a small sherry would be appropriate at bedtime. (You might need something yourself, and you know that a glass of wine a day is supposed to help delay dementia … so think of it as medicinal!)

● When you are at the end of your tether you may consider asking the doctor for a sedative. You have to be careful with them, though, because they can cause a 'hangover' the next day, when the person is drowsy and more likely to doze, and not take enough exercise or eat enough, which means there may be trouble the next night. If they are dopey it might cause a fall. However, needs must when things get tough.

My husband wakes up in the middle of the night craving a banana sandwich. Give him that and a slurp of milk and he will drop off to sleep again very quickly. He ought to brush his teeth, but who cares, if it is a choice between that and a better night's sleep for me? I make up the snack in advance to keep it quick and simple. (Wife of C., 62)

Wandering

In academic circles there are arguments about what to call 'wandering'. I use this word because it is probably the term that most people use and understand. The reason for wanting to use other words is that the person is not usually drifting around, but heading purposefully for something. Our problem is that we don't know what that purpose is, so it looks like pointless wandering. And even if we find out that the purpose is something futile, such as setting off for work decades after retirement, or popping round to see long-dead friends, or getting down to the school to collect the little ones, who are now grown up and living in New York, we can still do something that will help.

- Step one is to try to work out the purpose. You can gently or casually enquire about where they are going and what they are looking for and offer help. Start to get a picture of what's usually wanted and you can anticipate it. Maybe there is someone who will take them for a walk every morning right at the time they always want to leave the house? If you are busy and live near a dangerous road you will be tempted to lock the front door or the garden gate. The problem with this is that the person will probably redouble their efforts to get out and they'll become angry and frustrated – feelings that may be taken out on you. This is where being able to anticipate the problem and make a plan will help.

- Exercise is a magical solution to many problems. Whatever the reason for wanting to wander, a person is less likely to do it if they are physically tired. If they have an overwhelming sense that they want to go somewhere, then getting the right clothes and shoes on and getting someone to go with them is good. As people with dementia are often older and frailer, a diverting walk with an offer to return home for a cup of tea and a sit-down after is often enough to calm them and in the end takes up less time than arguing about it all day.

- The kinds of ideas that would give rise to anxiety and the need to get out are less likely to occur if the person with dementia is busy and occupied. Boredom and frustration go hand in hand. Your house is not a holiday camp and you need to do chores and live your own life, but planning for some distractions can be really helpful.

I got a box set of episodes of Cheers. *To be honest, I could have just bought one disc, because he is happy to watch it over and over. Just hearing the theme tune starting again is enough to get him to get into his chair and settle down. (Wife of Rex, 82)*

- When judging a Design Council competition I was introduced to the 'dementia dog'. This was originally thought of as a career-change opportunity for dogs who failed the practical at 'dogs for the blind' training. These companion animals are a great idea. The dog needs walking and wears a vest that tells the world that he is looking after his master. Unlike dogs for the blind, which have to be respected and not petted when they are working, this animal is an invitation to stop and talk.

They can also be trained to respond to a timer in the house by fetching a bag with medicine in when the timer goes off to remind you to take your medication. And if you give the order 'Home!' it can help overcome that problem of returning to the wrong house.

● There are a lot of assistive technologies available now that will let you know where the person is, even within their house, even if you can't see them or have gone out yourself. There has been bad publicity about them from time to time, equating them with the 'tagging' of criminals and ignoring the restriction of human rights through deprivation of liberty.

Dot Gibson, NPC [National Pensioners Convention] general secretary, said, '… This is trying to solve a human problem with technology. Rather than tagging people we need better social care out in the community. Dementia patients need human interaction not tagging. Using electronic tags on dementia sufferers raises very important issues about the individual's human rights. … Older people are effectively being demonised and treated like criminals.'

Neil Duncan-Jordan, national officer of the National Pensioners Convention, called the practice 'inhumane' and said, 'It smacks of criminality' and puts them 'on a par with common offenders or people with Asbos…

'There has got to be a more humane way of coping with somebody's mental state…' (www.homecare.co.uk)

To be honest there is nothing very liberating about being locked in because you are likely to stray, or dying in a ditch because you got lost and no one could find you.

● Years ago there was a community that created an 'organised wandering' system. It was relatively rural and (with the right permissions) as many people as possible were informed about the one or two men in the area who were likely to go for a walkabout and not find their way back. Each day they'd be provided with the right footwear and clothes and be let loose. Of course there were risks, but the risks of attempting to deprive them of their liberty by restraining them at home were also significant. They included the likelihood of the men being sedated, with all the side effects involved, and the possibility of them getting aggressive with those who wanted to keep them in. People guided them back, or went walking with them. These days there are sophisticated tracking devices that mean you'd always be able to find people, even if the community turned the other way and did not take care of them.

- You may have already had some narrow escapes. Part of your plan must be to make a list of the places where the person is likely to go. Your previous house, their favourite pub … you know their usual haunts. Research from search and rescue organisations emphasises that men and women have different wandering patterns. Men are more likely to go off the beaten track. Women are more likely to head for the shops. It sounds like a sexist cliché, but if it helps find them, who's complaining? If you have that horrible moment of panic when the person seems to have got lost, it is important that you are able to give the police or helpful neighbours the best possible description. Remembering what they were wearing is a good start, but a recent digital photo that can be quickly shared is useful. Take a new one frequently.

- Almost always the person is found. When that has happened you have to relax. You are doing the best that you can and you can't be criticised for it. Be careful not to make your home into a prison for yourself, because that is worse. You have your plan for this happening again and you will be even more efficient the next time. It's time to get that locator device.

Other difficult things

When someone has dementia you may reach a stage where you are more involved than you ever expected to be with their bodily functions. Problems with continence can be the last straw that causes someone to go to a care home because some people are unable to manage it. But with help, many can.

Incontinence is a bit of an issue but I've had two visits from the continence nurse and I've got a little routine sorted out. I treat him like a puppy. After each meal I take him to the toilet and sit him down and he usually does his business then. I only get soiled pants occasionally at night so the laundry isn't too awful. (Janice, wife of James, 81)

This gracious older lady is managing a difficult problem with an intensely practical and unemotional response. Whatever you might think about the way she describes it, she's doing an amazing job and keeping her husband where he will be best loved and looked after – at home. There is no point in entering into discussion with her about privacy or dignity. In the quiet of their own home she has found a solution that creates the right balance for them and she knows what she is doing.

There are practical issues for carers about how to wash 'faeces' (more commonly described as 'poo') or solid waste off sheets and blankets or take it off other furniture. It is unpleasant to think about, but the most important practical thing is to scrape off excess solids into the toilet and soak the bedding in a detergent that contains enzymes, before washing in hot water. You can be prepared by having cleaning gloves, disposable plastic bags and paper towels on hand, and the right detergent. There is a cheerful website called 'Housewife How-to's' that has even more advice in this line: housewifehowtos.com/clean/how-to-clean-poop/.

In the US there is a National Association for Continence (NAC), which says, 'Let's get past the embarrassment and on with our lives.' It reports that over twenty-five million Americans are affected by incontinence, but that successes are on the rise. In the organisation's really useful website, www.nafc.org, it talks about the fact that this is a really sensitive area, but it gives practical advice. There are also sites in the UK that can help and they are listed at the end of the book or can be found through the Association for Continence Advice.

While many of us could contemplate discussing some of the behavioural issues that arise, there are some relationship issues that are so personal, so taboo, that it is almost impossible to enter into discussion with anyone. This may be particularly difficult for older people, because we've not ever been allowed to talk much about relationships or sex to strangers.

He's stronger than me, and since this dementia set in, he's been a bit of a handful. He wants to go to bed with me three times a day for sex. It's as if he's forgotten about it immediately after. It is bad enough that he is so indiscreet about it, but these demands are too much. The nurse suggested distracting him but he gets aggressive if I refuse. (Eleanor, 79)

Changes in a couple's sex life are to be expected if one is ill and the other is exhausted with caring, but the hyperactivity described here is more akin to aggression and you would need professional help if it is a problem. Sexual hyperactivity is a problem which should be referred to the psychiatric service. Your safety and well-being should be the primary concern of your GP, but it may be that you also need to talk to a counselling organisation like Relate if you find it really hard to open up about the subject. You must be reassured, though, that this problem is not unheard of and there may be medication that can help.

Another area that causes disturbance is something doctors call 'repetitive vocalisation'.

I need help with dealing with repeated questions. It was suggested that I repeat the answer using the same words. But what if it gets asked again and again? It's all too easy to let the ... exasperation show. Sometimes I'd just end up saying, 'Oh, you know, I've forgotten,' and Mum would laugh (I'm not sure how comfortable a laugh that was though). (Ruth, whose mother had dementia)

This repetitive behaviour is one of the most annoying and intractable problems in dementia. No one knows what to do about it, apart from distraction. For a carer, being able to zone out is very good. Teenagers often seem to know how to say 'Uh-huh' at the right point in a conversation without actually being aware of or paying attention to what is being said to them. If we knew how they do that we could teach it to carers for selective use in times of desperation.

We know that disturbing behaviour in people with dementia is often a response to their misunderstanding and fear about what is happening to them. We can do a lot to reduce that behaviour by removing or changing the triggers. It is important to watch out for the way in which health and social care staff may set off the behaviour. You might think that these are people who should know better, but often they have not had any education in this area. The care worker who is accustomed to cheerfully and confidently walking into a stranger's house, undressing them and diving in and out of their rooms, moving and handling their possessions, is just doing her job. She assumes that her client has agreed to and even wants her services. But if her client has dementia they may not remember ever having agreed, so her 'normal' style is going to cause problems. If you have any control or influence at all, use it to indicate that you want staff to be not just 'dementia aware' but educated in how to manage dementia in a person's home. All your hard work should not be undone by people who are supposed to be helping.

Remember that what you are dealing with is very hard at times and make sure to give yourself a break.

Chapter 9

Your dementia-friendly home

By 'home' I mean the house or apartment where you live. This can be a place that you've lived in for a long time, or somewhere you've moved to in later years, or perhaps you have moved very recently to help deal with practical problems associated with dementia. Some of the ideas in this chapter are about changes that you can make now and others are things you could consider if you were moving to a new or purpose-built place. There are suggestions that are inexpensive and some that are fairly major, and you would not always do everything described here. For example, you would not change all the floor coverings in your house on the basis of this advice, but if you had decided to change them anyway you might consider these ideas when choosing your flooring.

My husband is a cabinetmaker and builder and although neither of us has dementia or anything like it, we make dementia-friendly decisions whenever we are making any change in our house. It all looks really nice, not like some of the ugly adaptations that you see. So even if he passes away before me, and I get dementia, he'll have made sure that I can stay in our house for longer. (Mrs C., 62)

If you or someone who lives with you has dementia you've got a lot on your plate. Some of the problems that occur every day can't be avoided, but some of them can. If you sort out the avoidable problems by making adjustments in your home, you can concentrate your energies on the issues that are more difficult to resolve.

General hints

- As with most of these hints, there are two routes here. In the person's own home change as little as possible apart from increasing the light and removing hazards. The only changes you should make are those that are really required for safety and security. If the person is moving, make things dementia-friendly. To be dementia-friendly everything should be 'obvious' – that is, it should be traditional in design.

- Remember that the person with dementia has difficulties with recall, working things out, learning new things and coping with disabilities or impairments, all of which is very stressful, so when you make any changes you have to keep this in mind.

- If you are staying in the old place, keep it the same. Decluttering is good if you can get away with it, but be aware that the person may turn round and ask for the object today that they asked you to throw away yesterday.

- If you move to a new place, remember to keep everything as obvious and familiar as possible. In some cases the dementia only really comes to light after a move. After a move the person may wake up in the morning, having forgotten that they've moved, and try to get back to the old place. This demonstrates that an unfamiliar environment can challenge someone who is having problems with working things out, learning new things and remembering.

- Make the place as stress-free as possible. There are more hints on this later in the chapter.

Light

Physiological changes in the eye mean that the capacity to see steadily deteriorates from a young age. By the time people are about 75 years old they need twice as much light as normal lighting standards recommend, and nearly four times as much as a 20-year-old, in order to see satisfactorily. The two implications ... are that twice the 'normal' light is required, and that the lighting level in spaces should be set by someone who is of mature years. (Dementia Services Development Centre)

- People with dementia are usually older, and the older we are the more likely it is that we will start to have impairments of eyesight. The lens, the clear part of the front of the eye, yellows over time, so it is as if the older person sees the world through a pair of yellow goggles that get thicker each year. Every old person needs to have more light to counteract this, but it is even more important if the person has dementia. In dementia the person finds it harder to remember where anything has been put, so having lots of light means they don't have to remember so much because they can see.

- Older eyes find it harder to adjust to changes in light levels, so if you have lights that switch on automatically with movement sensors, make sure that they go on earlier and stay on for longer than you instinctively feel is enough. When I'm headed up the stairs, it's no use if the light does not go on until I am at the first step, because I will be halfway up before my eyes have adjusted to the new light level. Watch out if the optician is trying to persuade your dad to have a photo-chromic tint on his bifocals. It is all very well trying to look like a Mafioso with shades on, but he might fall over when he steps back into the house from the sunlit garden.

- Energy-saving light bulbs will make a contribution to saving the planet, but if your dad was an early adopter of that technology he probably bought his a number of years ago, when they still had a problem with longevity. The newer light bulbs seem to last for ever compared with old-fashioned ones, but year on year they lose their luminosity.

We've got some of those energy-saving bulbs in our house that seem to suck light in rather than give any out. Time to 'fix' them even though they are not 'broken', in my view. You'd need a miner's lamp to get about the house. (C., daughter of Mr C., 63)

- The cheapest light comes through the windows. Get a curtain rail that allows the curtains to open right back to maximise the aperture. If the window faces a wall, paint the wall white so that light is reflected in. Cut back vegetation and clean the glass. You have to watch for glare, which is unhelpful, but there are ways of reducing that without reducing light: for example, using fine nets. Nets also help with the previously mentioned problem of windows behaving like mirrors at night. If the person sees their own reflection in the glass when it is dark, they may misinterpret what they see. Have the electric lights on all the time, with light sensors that just switch them off when the natural light reaches the required level.

- Daylight has the added advantage that it helps to set the body clock, the internal mechanism that makes you sleepy at night. Melatonin is the naturally occurring hormone that sets your body clock. International travellers buy it in tablet form to help them overcome jet lag. In your body the production of this useful molecule is reduced in old age and even further in dementia. It's one of the reasons that people with dementia turn night into day. Its metabolism is stimulated by daylight falling on the retina at the back of the eye, particularly the spectrum of light in the early part of the day. Getting out in daylight can really make it more likely that the person will sleep (there is more on this in the section about bedrooms: see page 189).

- If you are going to change one thing only, increase the number or strength of the light bulbs throughout the house. Avoid subtle or subdued lighting. More is better, but you must check the light fittings to make sure they are not being overloaded. If there is a pendant light in the room with three branches, get one with five.

- Some of the useful objects in the house need to be more obvious than before. If the person always had a bedside clock, get a bigger one and put it in exactly the same place. Make sure that their spectacles are up to date. Optometrists will come and see you at home very happily. In their offices they have equipment that will test for a range of eye problems and can often refer you directly to the eye hospital if there is a serious problem.

I dreaded her getting cataracts done when the optician said my mum needed it. Our grandmother had to lie still in hospital for days after when she had it. But it is ever so quick these days. It took about half an hour and we had to be careful for a day or two, but it got better really fast. It has given her a new lease of life. She started watching her films again and keeping herself occupied happily in the day. She was getting miserable before. (Daughter of D., 92)

Sound

Losing your hearing is a bit like going to a foreign country where you speak only a bit of the language. You struggle … and just trying to get by leaves you exhausted. This is exactly what happens to people who suffer hearing loss. As a result, they may start to withdraw from many of the activities they used to enjoy, because certain scenarios might tire them out, or might be embarrassing or difficult. Now we think this could have a worrying knock-on effect: evidence is emerging that deafness may lead to dementia ... Whether one is causing the other, or whether they're simply associated, is not clear. But we do know that deafness leads to a greater cognitive load. And if your brain has to make more of an effort to do one task, it will be compromised in others. (Professor David McAlpine, Director of the University College London Ear Institute, Mail Online, 12 March 2013)

- Remember that there is a difference between sound and noise. If you talk to someone who has had a hearing problem after they get a hearing aid they tell you that it's difficult at first. Everything is amplified, so the noise of, say, the air conditioning and traffic is as noticeable as the sound of voices in the room. They have a problem in differentiating between noise and meaningful sounds. People with dementia seem to have a similar problem. It's hard for anyone to concentrate if there are lots of distracting noises and they are tired. As this is what it is like when you have dementia, anything you can do in your house to minimise meaningless noise is very valuable. If you have an impaired capacity to think, you need all the help you can get.

- Having the TV or radio on when no one is watching or listening is an obvious issue. It only makes life difficult for the person with dementia. Music can help people to relax and that works best if it is their favourite music, so an iPod with personalised music tracks is ideal. It's better than listening to the radio, where music is often interrupted with commercial breaks, news or pointless chatter. Design the auditory environment so that you can get positive benefits from what the person can hear and eliminate the negative effect of communal undifferentiated noise.

A movie has been made to document the 'Music & Memory' project … familiar music from our youth is often untouched during the course of the disease. No matter the degree of memory loss, music has the power to help us feel whole, lift our mood, reduce anxiety, and help us feel more alive. Alive Inside: A Story of Music and Memory follows Dan Cohen, a social worker who decides on a whim to bring iPods to a nursing home. What Dan Cohen discovers by accident, and scientists have been studying for years, is that a person suffering from memory loss can seem to 'awaken' when given music they have an emotional attachment to. As Oliver Sacks explains, 'Music imprints itself on the brain deeper than any other human experience. Music evokes emotion and emotion can bring with it memory.' (Reported by Alzheimer's Disease International)

- Soft furnishings like carpets and curtains help to absorb noise. In the person's familiar surroundings you would want to change as little as possible, but this is worth remembering if you are moving to a new place or to live with a relative. The current fashion for wood-effect flooring is very practical and hygienic, but carpet tiles can give a high level of hygiene while reducing the clatter that comes from furniture scraping about and the noise of feet.

- Meaningless squeaks and clatters get magnified by hearing aids, so make sure that these are well maintained and that more than one person knows how to adjust them and replace the batteries. Controls can be very small and awkward. Get ears checked regularly. You must not assume that the person does not understand you because of their dementia when in fact they are just not hearing you because they need a nurse to syringe their ears.

- If you have good concentration you can ignore what is going on around about you. When concentration is difficult, extraneous noise makes life difficult, particularly if you are prone to misinterpreting noises because of cognitive impairment. Take time to sit in your house with your eyes closed and listen to the noises round about. See what you can do to reduce any of them.

- Studies show that people do not get themselves a hearing aid until years after they would benefit, so consider a test. People who lack their back teeth seem to risk a build-up of excess impacted earwax because its production and elimination are promoted by jaw movement. The local nurse may be able to syringe ears regularly if the doctor can see that sort of problem, which is increased by the use of hearing aids because they cause the wax to become impacted. Not all local practices offer syringing.

In medieval times they used earwax for the preparation of pigments for illuminated manuscripts. Now the doctor usually doesn't even check after syringing to see if it has been removed. It's worth asking for them to do that even if you are not going to make personal use of it! (Dementia nurse)

The latest research from the World Health Organization states that attending to hearing loss is one of the twelve evidence-based things you can do to delay cognitive impairment. The sooner the better.

Floor coverings

- There is evidence that a person with dementia will walk more swiftly and safely over a smooth, matt, unpatterned surface.

Being able to move about depends on a whole range of factors, including how fit you are, how mobile, what shoes you have on and whether you can see. Having the floor covering right is just one element. However, if being slow to get moving makes the difference between getting to the toilet in time and not, you can see the benefit in having the right flooring. Avoid patterns. No shiny walking surfaces. Have the floor contrasting with the walls and try to use the same colour throughout to avoid 'junctions' where one room colour meets another, which is made particularly difficult if there is an obvious threshold strip.

The interior designers for the new hospital fancied a floor pattern that divided the corridor flooring along the full length with two-thirds being darker than the other third – two shades of grey. We said that this would not be 'dementia-friendly' due to depth-perception problems. They ignored this. Now the nurses tell us that old people are falling over in those areas. (Dementia Services Development Centre [DSDC] design team leader)

- The changes in how well a person with dementia walks may be caused by the underlying disease, which leads to coordination difficulties in some cases. All of us stumble once in a while, but the danger with dementia is being slow to recover from a stumble and consequently falling. Trip hazards in the home may be really obvious and need to be dealt with as a matter of urgency. The community occupational therapist may be able to help with this, but mostly it is common sense. Imagine shuffling through the house, then check what would trip you, including door thresholds and little mats.

- Any hard surfaces, such as ramps indoors and out, and bathroom and kitchen floors, should be covered with one of the commercial non-slip floor coverings that are available. These should reduce the likelihood of a fall even if wet.

- The flooring usually stops at a skirting board where it meets the wall. Paint these boards a contrasting colour to the floor. Some people with depth-perception problems have difficulty in working out where this junction is, and this makes it hard to judge where you are putting your feet. For example, there is a fashion for taking the floor covering up the wall a few centimetres, which you often see in wet-rooms. This gives a visual illusion that the floor is a few centimetres higher than it is and the consequent misplacing of a foot when the person tries to step up on entering the room can cause them to stumble.

- The use of 'colour coding' in dementia does not help. This is where you try to orientate people by associating different areas with different colours.

They keep telling me I live in the blue corridor (or is it the green,..? I forget) but I wish they'd just put up a signpost! (Eleanor, 93)

The most important thing to say about floor coverings is that they should contrast with the walls.

Decoration and furniture

- If you are considering redecorating the place where someone has lived for a long time, ask yourself why. It could be that the turmoil makes it not worthwhile. Remember that just increasing the light is really helpful.

- For the training of health and social care staff one can buy spectacles that mimic a range of visual impairments, including those that are more common in older people with dementia. You want to check the environment? By wearing sunglasses smeared with petroleum jelly while trying to walk around the house, you can test the environment yourself for colour contrast, including noting the visibility of furniture, bedding and towels.

Contrast is the key to vision. If there is no contrast, objects cannot easily be seen and differentiated ... As we age we lose the ability to differentiate colours clearly, our perception of depth diminishes, there is a loss of visual acuity, we have less spatial awareness and our sensitivity to contrast lowers. Without good contrasts, the world becomes hazier, we struggle more and more to make sense of it and we function in life with less confidence. (DSDC Design Resource Centre)

- If you must do papering or painting, note that wall coverings with strong patterns can cause optical illusions for some people with dementia. It is worth keeping things simple, with bland colourings for most walls and a high degree of contrast between colours of doors, skirting boards and floors.

- Having increased the light level, use light paint on the ceiling and light-coloured curtains. Particularly after dark, the curtains and ceiling take up a lot of the person's field of vision, so make use of the opportunity to reflect light into the room from the curtains.

- I'm often asked about good colours and bad colours, and if they affect mood. There is no research evidence for mood alteration from colour in itself. However, someone like me might like Wedgwood blue because it reminds them of the walls in their childhood home. It might make them feel calm and safe. It's not an intrinsic quality of the colour that matters but rather the association.

- There is discussion about whether there is good or bad art for people with dementia. Again, this is a question of taste and association. As recent memories fade, the collection of graduation photos of my grandchildren might start to lose meaning, but a photo of my own mother's wedding day may mean a lot to me until I die. Some care homes go overboard with pictures of the local area in 'times gone by'. With the age range of residents being quite variable, and social and geographical mobility, this is often just a gimmick. It is nice and interesting, but it is not really related to dementia care.

- If you are inclined to forget where useful objects are, glass-fronted cupboards and wardrobes are available and chests of drawers with open fronts to let you see what is inside. Of course you could also label the drawers.

- Mirrors (and other reflective surfaces) cause practical problems. If you have forgotten the last twenty years and you see an eighty-year-old version of yourself in the mirror, you will be inclined to think that it's not you. You are expecting to see a much younger person. You may think that this is a stranger looking through a window. You can cover mirrors and pull curtains over reflective window surfaces to prevent this disconcerting experience.

One of our residents had become incontinent and demonstrated agitated behaviour when we attempted to escort her to her en suite shower room to use the toilet. She screamed and shouted and appeared to be saying that there was a 'devil' in there. We removed the mirror above the sink and she started to use the toilet normally again. (Care home supervisor)

Assistive technology

There is a wide range of technological solutions to some of the common problems that dementia brings. Some of these solutions have been mentioned elsewhere in the book. This technology can be used for safety, for locating people who might get lost, for entertainment and for distraction. New products continue to be developed all the time, so it is important to keep an eye out for the latest products. Prices come down all the time and your local authority may be prepared to bear some of the cost as part of their effort to keep people living in the community. Ask your local social services.

- If you are anxious about the person leaving the house and getting lost, you may wish to use a locator device. You can buy one that can be worn as a discreet wrist band like a watch. There are many commercial brands available, some of which include a facility to track your loved one by PC or smartphone. This has the advantage that you can allow or even encourage the person to go out and about, secure in the knowledge that you will be able to locate them if needed.

- Security of the home is an issue. The person may leave the house without locking it or lose keys. They may be anxious about too many keys circulating in the community: for example, if there are carers in and out of the house from time to time. A key safe is a small box fixed to the wall or the door handle in which a spare key can be stored and accessed only by using a secret combination. This means that legitimate visitors or carers can enter without anyone having to come to open the door, and the person does not need to worry about answering the door if there is an unexpected or nuisance caller. The biometric lock that has already been mentioned is commercially available and can store up to eighty fingerprints. This means that someone can open the door at a touch if they've been included on the list. The provision of an ordinary key and a combination lock makes secure access and door opening flexible for unexpected emergencies. It adds to safety because it locks automatically when the door is slammed shut, but can be opened from inside without a key at any time.

- Infrared-beam emitters are useful, light and easy to install. They can emit a beam which, when it is broken, will control lights as soon as the person enters or leaves an area. They can be used to warn the carer that the person is on the move. This can be via a buzzer under a sleeping carer's pillow or a signal on their mobile phone. You can also acquire an electronic monitoring system which involves very small wireless sensors being placed in the kitchen, bathroom, living room and bedroom to monitor the movement of the person around their house. A family member or carer can access this information via the internet and reassure themselves that the person with dementia is up and about and doing normal things.

I can log on to my laptop and see a chart of my dad's movements about the house. It showed him always to be getting up very early, so we arranged for home care before six a.m. To begin with he thought we were going to be filming him, but he now understands that there is no camera or sound, just a blip on a screen when movement happens in the room and that I don't look all the time, just a couple of times each day or when I think of it. One brilliant example is when the early-morning carer wondered if he was sleeping in the chair at night and not going to bed. The movement monitor proved he was going to bed. He just made the bed so neatly that it looked like it had not been slept in. (Andrew, talking about Douglas, 92)

- Safety is an issue in everyone's home. For people with dementia there is an additional problem, because relatives and the authorities may be very risk-averse. People forget that a person with dementia does have a right to do unwise things. Electronic monitoring actually helps give freedom to people with dementia because it reassures the relatives. Over-anxious relatives have in the past unnecessarily accelerated the date when someone has to leave their own home.

● All the ordinary accident-prevention strategies that are used
in everyone's home, including smoke and carbon monoxide
detectors, must be correctly installed, with working batteries
properly fitted or wired in. Cookers are a particular concern. It
is possible to arrange the hob so that the person in the house
cannot switch it on randomly and so that it always switches
itself off after a short period of use. Alarms such as heat alarms
have their place, but they are problematic if the person with
dementia does not understand the meaning of the noise when
the alarm sounds and fails to exit the house in an emergency.

● Medication alerts are among the personal electronic devices
that are useful in managing dementia.

*I've got two bits of kit I recommend. One is a pillbox. You have to
turn it upside down to take the pills out and when you do that an
electronic alert signal to your family (for example, your daughter, at
work in the city) is cancelled. If you don't knock out the pills at the
right time, she gets an alert advising her to phone you about it. The
second is a Magiplug. If you put the plug in the sink and turn on
the water, and then forget about it, the plug will automatically drain
the sink before it overflows. I give that one to students for Christmas.
(Dementia nurse)*

● It is vital to bear in mind that assistive technology is not
without its problems. It has to be acquired and maintained, and
people with dementia have to consent to its being used in their
own home. Some of the devices are possibly irritating or even
bewildering. If you have always lived alone, a voice coming
out of the partition asking you about your keys or if you
need help might be frightening rather than reassuring. Some
electronic inventions are dazzling, but they can only be one
part of the answer to the challenge of maintaining the dignity
and autonomy of the person with dementia. Fall detectors are

important, but if they are left dangling on the bedpost they don't help when the person falls on the stairs.

What to do in the bedroom

- Sleep is really important in dementia. The condition is crushingly tiring and so the person with dementia needs to rest. If they don't sleep at night it causes health and well-being problems for the people who live with them which are so serious that it can precipitate the person having to be admitted to hospital or a care home. The design of the bedroom can help. And of course you also need to think about all the common strategies, like plenty of exercise and daylight during the day, followed by a bedtime routine that involves winding down and perhaps having a warm drink (see Chapter 8 on sleeplessness).

- Bedrooms are for relaxing, sleeping and doing intimate things. It's best to keep entertaining and communication equipment such as televisions and computers elsewhere. There is increasing awareness that the light from screens falling on the retina affects the body clock negatively.

- People sleep best where it is dark and quiet and where the room is slightly cooler and the bed warm. From a practical point of view, how you achieve this depends on the design of your house and the time of year. Blackout curtains and blinds can help in summer.

- Put away daytime objects such as clothes to reduce the possibility of the person getting up and getting dressed for the day prematurely.

- The commonest reason for getting out of bed is to use the toilet. A commode is handy for people with restricted mobility, but when you've got dementia you might not recognise it for what it is, as it is an unfamiliar object that you'd have to learn to use.

● It is not usual to label drawers or put up signs, but it might just be that these things will help the person find what they want when they get up in the night.

● Get a full night's sleep yourself as a carer by using electronic equipment to monitor the person. You can relax, confident that if anything untoward happens you will soon know about it. Sleep deprivation in carers may have detrimental effects on your immune system, whether you have reduced quality or duration of sleep. Some people sleep better in bed beside their husband or wife with dementia. Others can only get a decent sleep if they move into another room. The emotional significance of such a move is not to be underestimated.

I bought my mum a baby alarm. It's the same model we use for our small children. She had been sleeping on the sofa downstairs beside Dad in case he needed her in the night. Now she can go up to bed and get a decent sleep. They both look better already. (Danielle, daughter)

Bathrooms and toilets

● Incontinence can be a problem in dementia, but it is not inevitable in everyone. In the early stages it is most likely to be caused by not being able to get to the toilet in time. The person might forget to go, or they might not leave enough time to get there and get out of their clothes. It's potentially embarrassing and inconvenient. In some cases it is caused by, or made worse because of, difficulty in finding and using the toilet. There is further discussion about various aspects of finding the toilet throughout the book.

- If your house is a perfect design there will be an en suite toilet in the bedroom in addition to a downstairs toilet for convenience. The en suite toilet will have the toilet pan positioned where it can be seen from the head of the bed, and you'll have a movement sensor that switches on the light when you get out of bed. The toilet seat colour will contrast with the floor, and walls and the rest of the bathroom furniture. That's the ideal, so that is what you should expect in a newly designed care home or specifically designed housing, but there are ways round that in your own home. There is a balance to be struck between having enough light to find the toilet and it being dark enough to promote good sleep. It depends on what the person is used to.

One inventor came to me with a prototype 'glow in the dark' luminous toilet seat. I didn't really think it was a great idea for dementia; it was too unfamiliar. (Dementia nurse)

- Mirrors can cause problems – particularly in the bathroom, where they are required for grooming – if the person does not recognise their face any more.

- Light should be bright, but avoid glare. Contrasting colours in grab rails, toilet seats, hand towels, etc. are really helpful for people to see. Shiny floors should be avoided as they appear wet and can make the area seem dangerous. Watch out for reflective and shiny surfaces, which can cause problems with glare or reflections that are not understood. It is not only mirrors that cause problems.

- Wash-hand basins and baths should have classic designs of taps (faucets) so that they are easy to recognise and to use.

In our local Harvey Nicks there is a gorgeous ladies' toilet but my problem is the fancy taps. I twist them this way and that, often with soapy hands, and I can't work out whether you are supposed to use it like a lever or a knob. They're a miracle of continental fashion and design but I can't work them. (Jane, 59)

● Bath and sink plugs can be replaced with Magiplugs to avoid flooding accidents. We've seen places where people are not allowed to have a plug for fear of causing an overflow of water on to the floor. This little product has a pressure sensor in it so that if the water gets too deep, it releases the water down the drain. Centrally control the maximum temperature for hot water to avoid scalding accidents.

● Sort out the lock on the door so that you will be able to get in if assistance is needed, and it might be that an outward-opening door would help with that as well. Contrasting colours for grab rails are important, and removing items such as toilet-roll holders if you suspect the person is using them as a grab rail.

Kitchens and dining rooms

● Good design of the kitchen and dining room is vital for a person with dementia because eating and drinking are especially important for their health. In other chapters you will see how failing to eat and drink properly can lead to health problems, such as infections, falls and confusion – any of which can result in an admission to hospital, from which the person never returns to their own home. It is crucial to adapt the kitchen to allow people with dementia to enjoy food as much as possible for as long as possible.

When I was training to be a nurse we were taught that dementia was a 'wasting disease' and people got 'cachexia', which meant they withered away and died. I realised later, to my horror, that the main problem was that they never got enough to eat. (Jane, 59)

● Your aim should be that the person is able to continue to make meals for themselves and visitors for as long as possible, even if they are quite simple meals. When a person with dementia goes into hospital, they may have to undertake a kitchen assessment before they are 'allowed' to go home by the health and social care system. It's often undertaken by an occupational therapist. The sooner the dementia-friendly ideas are incorporated in their own kitchen the better. This will allow any of us to become used to our dementia-friendly kitchen before it is too late. The design of the kitchen can help you pass the test.

● There are design features that will encourage eating and drinking. These could include having a glass-fronted fridge so that all the tasty things are on view, or glass-fronted cupboards where the bright and attractive packaging of all the nutritious items is visible.

I find the secret is to do the opposite of what the slimming magazines recommend. They suggest keeping fattening foods out of sight. I recommend keeping them in full view – creating temptation. (Ellen, dietician)

● You can also use a little plug-in electric machine called an Ode, which will release at carefully timed intervals selected food odours that have been shown to make people hungry and more interested in eating. Combine this with the glass-fronted fridge that allows the person with dementia to see tasty treats and helps tempt them to eat. The glass door also makes it easier for a family member or carer keeping a stock check in case food is going off and needs clearing out. You might find such fridges marketed as wine coolers in the shops – just get different shelves.

● Keeping people involved with cooking is a good way of encouraging them to eat. You have to be sure that health and safety and food hygiene concerns don't take precedence over normal living. Careful planning helps, and looking out for the available assistive technology, such as microwaves with barcode readers so you don't have to read the print on the packaging, which is always too small. Another useful device is the induction hob that remains cool to the touch while heating up the cooking pan, and most of these induction units have safety functions that will shut them off if the pan is empty or there is no appropriate pan on the hob.

- You need to consider all the issues outlined elsewhere in this book about flooring and lighting when designing the kitchen. As ever, keeping the lighting bright is important. Trip hazards need to be considered and floor colours and coverings that support safe walking are needed. There are commercially available floor coverings that are easy to clean and will retain a high level of slip resistance even when wet and others that are frankly risky. Carpet may be hard to clean in the kitchen but it does have the advantage of being softer in the case of falls. Cleanable carpets and replaceable carpet tiles offer practical solutions. Remember that the culprit in the fall is often the footwear as much as the floor.

- Total risk-avoidance is seriously limiting, but often kitchen risks can be reduced by the use of technology. There needs to be a serious discussion about what level of risk is acceptable and to whom, as the estimation of the risk seems to vary hugely between hospital-based and community-based professional staff, with hospital staff having a bias against the person's own home. There are devices on the market that may reassure anxious relatives and neighbours who are afraid of accidents and falls. It is important to emphasise the right of the person with dementia to choose to take risks and not be deprived of their liberty. When the point is reached where the stove cannot be used safely, disconnect it, or remove the knobs if knob covers are not available. This is preferable to moving the person out of their home.

- Declutter the kitchen and put away things that are not often used, leaving out the stuff that is most likely to be used regularly, such as the kettle, tea bags and biscuit tin. Keeping things handy will discourage people from climbing on the furniture to reach high cupboards. Consider taking the doors off the front of some cupboard units or fitting glass doors so that contents can be found without too much searching. Anything that is out of the way is less likely to be used (appropriately or inappropriately). Remember the declutter/forgetting problem and be prepared to handle questions or confusion about where possessions have gone. Anything that is poisonous and could cause harm could be removed altogether.

- When appliances need to be replaced, buy the same brand and model if possible to help the person to continue to be able to use it. Keep the electric kettle away from the stove to reduce the chance of the person putting it on the hob by mistake. The first time that happens, get rid of it and buy a hob kettle. A whistle is needed if there is no automatic cut-off.

Living areas

- Internal spaces like living rooms, halls and stairs present their own challenges. People with dementia will be moving round the house with a variety of purposes, sometimes at night when they are tired and sleepy. Sometimes there will be a sense of urgency, as when they are going to the toilet. Worn or loose carpets have to be dealt with and banisters are best if they are on both sides of the stairs. People make mistakes about where the edges of furniture are, so sharp corners on furniture could be sanded down. Low coffee tables can be tricky.

● Lighting and light switches can help here. The light switches should contrast markedly with the wall to make finding easier. If the person has lived in the house for a long time, they may reach for the light switch without even looking, so this advice is even more important for custom-built supportive housing. You can make a significant improvement in visibility by changing the base plate of the switch or by framing it on the wall with some brightly coloured tape or other contrasting decorative material.

● The general principles about contrasting furniture and contrasts between walls and flooring that are described in other sections also apply here.

Outdoors

They offered us a place in a day centre, but what Dad really wanted was a buddy to take him up to the allotment and back; who would keep quiet and leave him in peace while he was there. (Daughter of J., 82)

● Going outside is really important for people with dementia. Chapter 8 explains how important exercise and exposure to daylight are for mood and sleep. There is a clear connection between vitamin D and falls, and the best source of vitamin D is sunlight on skin. Setting the body clock is only one of the benefits of getting outside.

● Pottering in the garden is a great way to stay well. Even if you don't have a garden you can get a great deal of pleasure from a balcony with pot plants on it, and a chair on which to sit and look out. A balcony is not automatically dangerous for a person with dementia, depending on what they are used to and the design of the balcony.

- If the family is concerned about the person with dementia leaving the garden and getting lost, it is possible to reduce the risk by having the right sort of fence or boundary. The gate in the fence can be made unobtrusive with planting or by putting the fastenings on the outside. It is also possible to put a fence halfway across the garden so that the person does have a gate that they can go in and out of at will.

- The garden is a great way of distracting people who may be agitated or distressed, because there is always something to do, whether it is weeding, sweeping paths, digging, grass cutting or even hanging out the washing. It offers additional benefits because the skills used outside have been there for a long time. There is great satisfaction to be had in showing young people how to do something like potting up a plant or taking a cutting.

To forget how to dig the earth and to tend the soil is to forget ourselves. (Mahatma Gandhi)

Chapter 10

What you should expect from the social care system

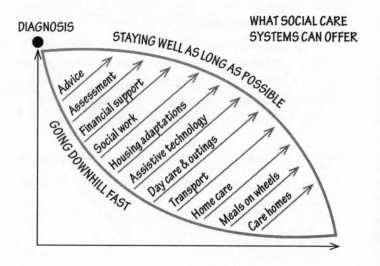

DIAGNOSIS

WHAT SOCIAL CARE
SYSTEMS CAN OFFER

STAYING WELL AS LONG AS POSSIBLE

GOING DOWNHILL FAST

Advice
Assessment
Financial support
Social work
Housing adaptations
Assistive technology
Day care & outings
Transport
Home care
Meals on wheels
Care homes

There is a wide range of social services to help people with dementia, although local availability and costs differ. This chapter explains how the social care system responds to dementia. The central regulation is clear. The government guidance says that if you are diagnosed with dementia, your future social care needs will be assessed and a care plan will be drawn up. Your carer is also entitled to an assessment. The social and personal care part of what you need is expected to come from the social services or social care department of your local authority or council and the health part from the NHS. The terms 'local authority' and 'council' are used to mean the same thing. This chapter explores what you can expect from them.

The question of what is a 'health' need and what is a 'social' need is sometimes a matter for debate. You may have to pay for all or some of the help arranged by social services, depending on your income and savings, while the NHS care you receive will largely be free. That is why the distinction between health and social care can act as a barrier to receiving services. It is an artificial distinction and not based on any logic or standard. In some places certain types of help are not available through the council even if you can pay. In these cases you need to search for private services, which can be of a very high standard and cost-effective, and may be provided by a 'community interest company' or 'social enterprise' or a voluntary organisation or charity. Although they are businesslike and take a payment, they do not make profits. Commercial companies may also offer high standards and good value for money. In every case you need to examine what is on offer and make up your own mind.

How the council and health services are divided up depends on local budgets and local systems. In some areas an occupational therapist will work for the council and in other areas for the health system. Both do the same kind of work, but the money for them comes out of different budgets that are decided by different people. This leads to variations in provision. One might have to be paid for by you and the other not. The situation is often described as a postcode lottery, but that's the price of local democracy. Whatever else you do, you have to be persistent to get what you want and perhaps be prepared to pay.

The process differs depending on whether or not the person is in hospital at the time they need an assessment. Patients sometimes find themselves trapped in hospital, waiting for a 'social work', 'social care' or 'community care' assessment (they unhelpfully give it different names, even in the same breath and even though it's the same thing). Occupational therapists do something called a 'home assessment', which should not be confused with a community care assessment. It is in fact one element of the 'community care' assessment. This can be frustrating for families who are dependent on assessments before the next step can take place.

Dad wanted to leave the hospital and we wanted him out of there because they were doing nothing. Medical care was completed and he was getting more agitated and depressed. We could pay for respite in a care home near his house. The staff nurse said emphatically that he could not leave until he'd had a social work assessment and the person who should do it was on her honeymoon. (That put me in a position where I knew more about her social circumstances than I needed.) He actually used the phrase that I was not 'allowed' to take Dad away. I asked him if this was a place of detention. It's mad. Everyone knows they are desperate for hospital beds and Dad was stuck because this social worker got married. (Eric, businessman, son of 83-year-old man with dementia)

Sometimes social care assessments are done by phone, at a day centre or in offices, but they are best done at home. Even if the person with dementia is in hospital, it is good to do part of the assessment at home. It is the capacity of the person with dementia and their carers to survive at home that is the crucial measure of what is needed.

Take a deep breath and accept all the help you can get with finding out what is on offer and what you are entitled to. A guide like this can only go so far, because there are over 300 local authorities in England alone, each with their own local rules and regulations. In Scotland there is some uniformity across the thirty-plus different organisations. Scotland has some national agreements on things like the amount that care homes will get paid from the public purse. But there are still differences, depending on the council. Wales and Northern Ireland are different again. And of course everything changes over time, sometimes quite rapidly.

The professionals and organisations that you are in touch with don't always communicate with each other as well as they should, and you will almost certainly find that you have to explain the situation each time you meet a new professional. Keep copies of forms and letters and a record of who you've seen, as it will help you to keep track and be useful for briefing the subsequent health and social care professionals you meet.

We had a visit from two original people from the council when she was first diagnosed but I've lost count now. They've got our records but I have to start from scratch explaining again every time. I used to object but one of them told me she can't rely on the others to have written it down right so I suppose it is better to keep telling them. They don't trust each other. (Daniel, husband, 75)

There are independent people who can help with finding a way through this maze. Remember the local Citizens Advice Bureau, because the more local your informant, the more relevant the information is likely to be. Age UK has some particularly helpful fact sheets, which have the advantage of being frequently updated. Their Fact Sheet 41 on local assessment is the best I have seen, but be warned: it is fifty-three pages long. When reading anyone's fact sheets online, be careful to check if they are describing what happens in England, Wales, Scotland or Northern Ireland in case you are tripped up by the differences. The internet is a blessing, but only if you remember to check that you are the intended audience for what you are reading. In general, if you are in England you have the least to worry about, because the default position tends to be that the service on offer and the person making the enquiry are both in England. The Alzheimer's Society covers England, Northern Ireland and Wales (not Scotland). Age UK covers England (not Northern Ireland, Wales or Scotland). Some organisations are really UK-wide: for example, the United Kingdom Homecare Association. Just check.

The council should be able to tell you:

- who is eligible to be assessed;
- how the assessor will decide what services will be provided;
- how and when to apply;
- how long you might have to wait for the assessment;
- which needs the local authority has said it will be able to meet;
- how to make a complaint.

In addition to the council, you can also get information on how to apply from the GP's surgery, the library or a local voluntary organisation like Age UK. Bear in mind that if you are doing this for someone else, they might refuse the assessment or the help that you have worked so hard to find. It's their choice.

I've seen my mother going downhill for months, and the GP did help by telling me how to get an assessment from social services. But Mother won't let them in the house. (Molly, daughter of 70-year-old woman)

If they are allowed over the threshold, social services will make their assessment of what seems to be the problem, and then decide whether or not to provide the services, and give a plan of how much they will provide and tell you how much that is going to cost.

What can you ask for?

You can only really demand an assessment. It's called a 'community care' assessment. Some local authorities do simple assessments on the phone and you would be right to be anxious in case these phone interviews are a form of rationing. A phone consultation is fine if the person on the other end is properly qualified to understand the issues, and if they are the sort of person who can explain processes and entitlements and options. For this reason, the person who does it (usually called a 'care manager') should be a qualified social worker or occupational therapist. If it is an assistant or student they must be under close supervision of the social worker who is taking professional responsibility for the case. It should not be an automated screening process by an administrator with a checklist. The quality of the response of the first contact is crucial and you should not hesitate to question or complain if you think you are being fobbed off. It is OK for them to warn you that you might have to pay, but you should not be put off having the assessment because of this.

Sometimes people get annoyed with the assessments. You may be asked all sorts of questions about all sorts of needs, when it turns out there were only ever a few services on offer, so most of the questions were irrelevant from your own point of view. The local authority has the power to decide what it will and will not provide, although it is required to take certain things into account when reaching a decision, and the government issues guidance on this from time to time. This is the government's way of trying to minimise the local variations that councils are otherwise entitled to make.

A person with dementia can refer himself or herself for an assessment. Alternatively a carer, friend or family member or the GP can make the referral, but only with permission, unless the person is so unwell with dementia that they have lost the capacity to make a decision like this. You can get the assessment no matter what your financial position. The money issue only comes in when the council is considering whether or not to charge for the services that it has assessed you as needing.

The social services staff will do a means test. This financial assessment will establish how much you'll have to contribute to the cost of providing services (if they offer them and you choose to accept). You are entitled to an assessment even if you are so rich that the local authority is unlikely to pay for anything you are judged to need. It is still worth undergoing this assessment because it gives you some guidance as to what there is out there that might help you, even if you are going to have to pay for it. And your circumstances might change. Carers are also entitled to an assessment, independent of the assessment of the person cared for.

Nothing is going to happen very fast unless it is an emergency. In England there is a twenty-eight-day target for assessments and another twenty-eight-day target for putting services in place. Even if a council is meeting those targets that whole process can take a couple of months. It is worth starting early, because you can always ask for a reassessment if the situation changes. A care and support plan is produced and the client or carers get a copy of it. It says what services the social services department thinks you need and how they'll be arranged.

It should contain:

- a note of the eligible needs;
- agreed outcomes and how the department will support them;
- a risk assessment, with actions;
- contingency plans for emergency changes;
- details of financial contributions that the person has been assessed to pay;

- support that carers and others have said they are willing and able to provide;
- support to be provided to the carer, as identified by their assessment;
- a review date.

If social services staff are really worried they have a legal right (and a responsibility) to put in an emergency service even before they've done a full assessment and made a plan. That's a good thing, usually. The plan should be reviewed within three months of the start and then at least once a year after. But you can ask for a review if anything changes. Sometimes budget changes mean that services that social work once provided free start to be charged for and some services are reduced or not provided at all any more. You can appeal, but that does not always make a difference (there is more about this in Chapter 15). If the local authority is not meeting their targets you can complain to the Local Government Ombudsman.

Because the government wants people to have choice and control over what happens, they are encouraging 'supported self-assessment'. In preparation, it is important to make a list of all the things that are a problem. Don't limit yourself to what is covered on any form they give you. It's worth keeping a diary so you can remember what problems occur from time to time that you might otherwise forget. The assessment should not assume that any carer is going to provide support. It might be that after discussion you agree to this, but it used to be that you would have a small chance of support if you had family around, as daughters will attest. There is also the problem that the assessment could consist of asking you only if you need the services that they know are on offer.

When Dad did leave the hospital, he needed some help to do his shopping so that he could continue to cook for himself. I was horrified to discover that he'd been put down for meals on wheels. He doesn't eat them, and he still was having problems with shopping. I started doing supermarket orders for him online; even though I live abroad, I can do that. (Daughter)

On the other hand, it is one better than asking you all about your needs and then *still* only offering you what they've got. Another issue is when you don't feel that you have a need, but the assessor thinks you are taking a risk. They have a duty to manage risk, but you have a human right, even if you are very old and have dementia, to make unwise choices. The balance between your autonomy and their risk management is a tricky one.

In England there are four levels of social service need defined by government guidance. These are Low, Moderate, Substantial and Critical. The council can choose which ones to fund, but they can't fiddle with the criteria as defined. Many have set their local funding bar at Substantial and Critical, so any needs below that are not met by them. Some even limit provision to Critical. Once they have set the bar, they can't use subsequent lack of resources as a reason to refuse support. Each authority sets its own eligibility bar, and if your needs meet those criteria you have 'eligible needs' and the authority has a duty to provide services for you. Authorities review the eligibility bar once a year, so they might decide from a particular date that they can only afford to fund Critical, where they once did both Substantial and Critical. If that happens you may find you are no longer eligible to receive something you used to have for nothing or at a reduced cost.

If public funds are not available for the social care you want from social services, there might be other public services that can help.

When I was looking for a home adaptation the social care assessment seemed to show I was not eligible, but housing put it in for me. They seemed to have another reason … maybe budget? I only thought to ask them when my cousin told me she had it from housing. It is bizarre, because this is all the same council. (Agnes, carer for her mother)

What might be on offer from social services?

In each of the four countries of the UK, what is potentially on offer is similar. For example:

- **Advice and information** about services and welfare benefits may be available through local authority websites, which are improving hugely all the time.
- **Community transport** – that is, accessible and affordable passenger transport services and includes dial-a-journey, taxi-card schemes and shop mobility.
- **Home adaptations** are commonly available. The physiotherapist or the occupational therapist often makes the decision on provision, and can also advise on things that you might buy for yourself. See Chapter 9 for design changes in the home.
- **Aids and equipment** These vary a lot and new things come on the market all the time. You sometimes don't know what you need till you see what there is … check out websites such as www.atdementia.org.uk for devices that will help with communication, leisure, safety, and prompts and reminders for people with memory problems. The local authority occupational therapist should advise on this.
- **Home meals or 'Meals on Wheels'** This is a service for people who find it difficult to access a hot meal or to cook

for themselves. Frozen meals are delivered, for example, on a fortnightly basis. If support with food preparation is needed a care worker can prepare meals and snacks for you. If you do not qualify for support, you can buy this service from the supplier yourself.

- **Day care** or the provision of safe, supervised care outside the home during the day may be on offer, for social contact and stimulation, in order to alleviate the responsibilities of a carer, while hopefully promoting independence in the person with dementia.

  Sometimes the transport arrangements are so bad that they undo a lot of the benefits.

- **Night-sitting** This is when someone comes to the house to allow the carer to get a full night's sleep. It can have a very positive effect on mental health.

- **Respite** This is often thought of as taking the person with dementia away somewhere to give the carer a rest, but more imaginative models now exist where the respite service is offered at home, so the person doesn't have to move and the carer can get away.

- **Help in placement in supported housing** This comes from social services. Sheltered housing may have thirty or forty self-contained units of accommodation with warden support and communal facilities like a laundry or a dining room. Each unit has a call system so that the resident can call for help to a warden who lives on the premises or to a call centre in case of emergency.

- **Care in a care home** If you need this, social services are responsible for arranging it. For self-funders (those who have to pay because their capital is over the charging limit) the council are only responsible for arranging it if the person is incapable of doing it themselves and has no family or friends to support them. There is much more detail about this in the companion, *Care Homes: The One-Stop Guide*.

Services to meet psychological, social and cultural needs

These should be provided but are often first in line for cutbacks when social care budgets are restricted. Loneliness and isolation have complex causes, but giving targeted support to those disproportionately affected, such as people who are widowed or physically isolated, or those who've stopped driving, is very important. Low-level telephone support is surprisingly effective.

Local authorities sometimes employ their own staff or give a contract to a voluntary or private organisation to provide these services. Giving work out to someone else is done on a competitive-tender basis, which is aimed at keeping costs down. Some people think that this is the explanation for any quality problems with what a council provides. Voluntary organisations may feel that they are subsidising the council, because they have so many donations of time and money that underwrite the services they provide in exchange for council grants. Charities may feel that they are being used as cheap labour in the name of community involvement. They even compete with each other for these contracts in the quasi-commercial process that is created by tendering. A tender is like a Dutch auction, where the lowest bid wins the contract. Quality is meant to be taken into account, but it is hard to measure quality in a proposed service. It's only when it is running that anyone really knows whether it can be done for that money.

Personal budgets (also known as self-directed support) and direct payments

With 'personal budgets', instead of being given a care plan setting out what social services have arranged for you, there is an allocation of money against your name that you control. You don't get cash, but a notional amount is set aside in the council's finance system that matches the cost of your assessed need. It is based on the estimate of what it would cost to give you what you'd have got from them under the conventional system. Instead of receiving the services they've decided for you, you can choose how you draw upon those services yourself up to the equivalent value from the council. You can work this out by talking to someone from the council or you can have an independent person called a 'broker'. The broker is often a local community organisation and may charge you for this service. This gives the person more choice over what is done with resources that are devoted to them, but it does not alter the amount of the resources.

As a slightly more daring alternative, the council can provide real cash for you to buy your own community care services from whomsoever you want. This is called 'direct payments'. In most cases councils are *required* to offer you this option, but it does not get taken up as much as one might imagine. If the offer comes from an official sucking their teeth and shaking their head over how difficult it is and how vulnerable you'd be if you made a mistake with the money, it is no wonder people don't take it up. There is some evidence that direct payments work well when people are supported to use them, but if the social work staff are cynical about them, the system is flawed. Also if social workers are under pressure and are accustomed to offering only what the system can offer, it is likely that people will get only what they've always been offered.

The system only provides an indicative figure of how much

services would cost, so the figure needs to be tested. At the very least the social work department should tell you how many hours of care they think you'll get for that amount and what the hourly rate is meant to be.

I used Dad's self-directed support money to buy short breaks for him (and us!) in the house of a family that lived near us. It started with them coming to look after him at our house, but he was just as happy going to them. (Daughter of Ahmed, 79)

Some people are put off the idea of buying the services they need directly. If you've never employed someone, it can be daunting. On the other hand, there is a legal requirement to make direct payments available to you if you want them. There is a perverse disincentive for council staff to recommend this. It's giving away their jobs. But the control you get is fantastic, as opposed to just having to take what's given. There is help and advice on becoming an employer available from Carers UK, which has a good quick guide (www.carersuk.org/help-and-advice/practical-help/care-and-support/direct-payments/direct-payment-quick-guide). There is also a website for Self Directed Support at selfdirect-edsupportscotland.org.uk and one called In Control (www.in-control.org.uk/about-us.aspx) which is a charity.

You want to avoid the pitfalls of having little or no control over the service you receive.

The wife of a retired chartered accountant with dementia said, 'I just started taking note of the names so I could remember properly and put a face to a name. Then each time a new face came so I kept writing, writing, writing, until we're here where we are today with 106 carers.' Two carers came four times a day, and his care was funded by social services. She said that her husband was an intensely private man but scores of strangers saw him naked. (Age UK worker)

If you need a lot of care, it might be cheaper for the council to place you in a care home rather than letting you stay in your own home. Some local authorities actually set a limit to the amount they will spend on care at home.

You probably already know your local authority. If you need to find them try this website: www.gov.uk/find-your-local-council.

Home care people

Having someone who comes into the house to help with care can be important. You may be able to get paid care workers known as 'home helps', 'home care workers' or 'domiciliary care workers'. Home care workers can also be known as 'care attendants' or 'personal assistants'. These people have a lot of different titles but generally provide practical support to help you to continue to care for the person you're looking after or to look after yourself in your own home. Some local authorities only fund home help in exceptional circumstances. You can buy it privately if you have the means, either by paying someone directly or using an agency.

Home help can provide services such as:

- 'domiciliary' care for the person you're looking after – this includes help with getting up and going to bed, bathing, dressing, meals and medication;
- help with shopping;
- helping the person you're looking after to go to the cinema, pub, shopping or to enjoy any other community activity;
- practical tasks around the home, such as cleaning and cooking;
- sitting with the person you're looking after to allow you to have a break.

You can employ someone directly yourself or use an agency.

If you use a private agency, they will provide a service through a team of care workers, which means you may not always have the same person visiting your home. The agency is responsible for training them. As a business, the agency will do its best to take your choices into account. You can sack them if they don't – unlike the local authority provision, where you mainly have to take what is provided. Local authorities also use teams, but you may have less power in influencing them because you are not the person paying.

Agencies are regulated: in England by the Care Quality Commission (CQC), in Scotland by the Care Inspectorate, in Northern Ireland by the Regulation and Quality Improvement Authority (RQIA) and in Wales by the Care and Social Service Inspectorate Wales (CSSIW). Agencies offer an advantage over you directly employing someone as they deal with complexities like payroll, training, disciplinary issues and insurance. They also replace workers when they are ill, on holiday or resign, and they should put things right when they go wrong. They vet workers before employment by taking up references and carrying out criminal-record checks on potential employees. They should train their workforce through induction, national qualifications and service-specific training.

You can find an agency by visiting the website of UKHCA – the United Kingdom Homecare Association (www.ukhca.co.uk).

Care in a care home

It used to be that care homes were retirement homes for relatively active people who could not or would not care for themselves. In general now between 70 and 90 per cent of care home residents have dementia, and the average length of stay in parts of the UK is eighteen months. So the care home is more often like a hospice for people with dementia and very frail people at the end of their life.

The local authority has to provide permanent care in a home for you if they have assessed you as needing this. You must have reached the stage where you cannot reasonably be supported to live in your own home. If you have no resources, they will pay for a standard care home place. Someone can add to that if they wish.

My mum is in a nice care home paid for by the council. She's got no money because Mum and Dad always lived in a council house and she never worked. I saw that they've got a lovely room overlooking the river with a balcony and much more space including an en suite bathroom. She loves a bath. We've got plenty of money since Don got this new job, so I'm paying extra to let her have the better room. (Jane, daughter)

If you have capital or income you have to pay. If you can't pay the cost from income because the fees are higher than your income, you have to use your own capital to pay for care. Even if you have enough money to go private, the council must organise it for you if there is no one in the family willing to do so and you are not able to do it yourself. They can't make your relatives do it.

If you are receiving financial support for the standard care home place and a relative or friend is happy to pay something, they can 'top up' the weekly payment to get you a better room or service. Unfortunately, it appears that such fees are being extorted from families who are told that no 'standard' places are available. It is worth challenging this position.

There is a scandal brewing about the fact that some local authorities in England never give enough money to the 'poorer' resident to pay for care, so that families almost always have to pay some extra money to get a care home room at all.

The council told us what rate they'd pay for Auntie Doris to go in a home, but there was not a single local care home that would take her for that amount. We had to chip in to top up her weekly rate. We are taking the council to court over it. We think they are in cahoots with the care homes. (Gordon, nephew)

For people living in Scotland there is a website called Care Information Scotland which has information on paying care home fees (www.careinfoscotland.co.uk/how-do-i-pay-for-care/paying-care-home-fees.aspx).

All the advice you can read on this is rather complicated and even if you find a helpful social worker they will tell you that it is hard to explain. If you have enough money you have to pay for your own care home care. That is called 'self-funding'. If you are self-funding in a care home, you are paying for your board and lodging, as you would in your own home. But you might need health care, such as help from a nurse. The home should not charge you for nursing if they provide it. The NHS should pay the care home for any health care you need from a registered nurse. They will make that payment to the home and you don't have to pay. The reason is this. The NHS is free and you should not have to pay for it just because you've moved out of your house. You could choose to have private health care, but that is a separate matter. Your care home can't bill you for it, because they can source the nursing for you from the NHS or get money for the nursing from the NHS.

In some circumstances there can be matters for debate about location. For example, if your old house was in one council area and your care home is in another, there is discussion about where you are regarded as 'living'. If one council or another does not wish to take responsibility for the cost of your care there could be a row.

Mum lived all her life in the council area next along from me and then when she got dementia we got her moved into a home in the council area where I live. My council says they won't pay for her because she's not one of their residents, and the other council say they won't pay because she's moved away. (Daughter of Imogen, 72)

It is not unknown for local authorities to argue over who has to pay but they can't delay services while they are working this out. See Chapter 14 for details about what to look for in a care home and remember that it matters which council area the home is in. Carers Direct can help you in England (tel. 0300 123 1053).

It drives me to distraction. All the old people want to come here to live and our local taxpayers are carrying the cost of caring for them when they need a care home. It's not fair. (Borough councillor)

NHS continuing care and joint packages of care

NHS continuing care is the name given to care that is arranged and funded by the NHS (not the local authority or a charity) for people who are not in hospital but whose dementia is very complex, or is complicated by other ongoing health care needs. You can get it in your own home or in a care home. It is different from NHS-funded nursing care, which may be given to you in your care home (as described above). NHS continuing care is different.

There is something else again called a 'joint package of care', which is where the local authority picks up the tab for your care but the NHS delivers the health part. The local authority part attracts a charge to you, but the NHS part does not. The NHS and the local authorities have different commissioning and procurement arrangements all over England, so the fear is that a failure to get on and manage those differences might lead to delays in some cases. There is more about NHS continuing care in Chapter 11.

Why are people anxious about social workers?

Britain has around two million people in the social care workforce. These professionals are under great pressure with cutbacks in funding and stress at work. They spend their days helping the most complex, needy and sometimes ungrateful people in our society. They are at the front line of explaining why benefits and services that everyone has come to expect will not be available. What they do is amazing and brilliant, most of the time. Research carried out by Age UK and the College of Social Work revealed in 2013 that over a quarter of all social workers resort to lying on official forms to get care for older people. This is against a background where they describe pressure to manipulate their assessments to avoid finding that people qualify for care. You would think that no one in their right mind would do this job. Many social workers regard it as a privilege to be involved in the lives of their clients and their families and derive great personal satisfaction from a good placement in a care home, or the resolution of a complex dementia problem. But you can't trust the system blindly. Understanding the system and knowing about local advocacy organisations may not turn out to be necessary, but it is worth having the information in case.

An 85-year-old dementia sufferer was 'kidnapped' by Essex County Council's social services department ... 'by this time we had been handed over to a third social worker ... By Monday we were on social

*worker number four' … fought for nine days to bring Enid Parkinson
home after she was taken into care – only achieving their goal after the
intervention of local government secretary Eric Pickles …*

*'I broke down in floods of tears … Finally she was safe, finally
she was away from social services, finally she was back in our care.'*
(Brentwood Gazette, 11 July 2013)

Social workers do not enjoy a good press, which is often unfair.
In this typical story their service is represented as fragmented and
arbitrary in its decision-making. But it is not only social workers
who are thought to fail people with dementia. Families are also
accused of this. There are even semi-professional groups set
up outside of social services to 'protect' people with dementia
against unfair treatment.

So what you need to do is understand dementia, take control
of the situation and work with the social work team, being clear
what your own aim is. Be politely determined about what you
believe you are entitled to and use the support of some of the
organisations listed at the end of the book, such as your local
Alzheimer's organisation.

*Recently I talked with an older man in a rural area who is working
out how best to support his mum in a city. He has been told by the
warden of her sheltered accommodation that she needs to be in a
home. He is 160 miles away from her, picking his way through lists
of contacts, information, forms and officials, plus doing his best to
support her. Getting the right care at the right time and knowing how
much it will cost and who should pay is like walking through treacle.*
(Sonia Mangan, Age UK)

Chapter 11

What you should expect from the NHS

When you are living with dementia it is really important to make the best of things, and the support that the health system gives you is a major element of this. In an ideal world, the health and social care systems would be so intimately linked that there would not need to be separate chapters on health and social services in this book. The reality is that services meant for one person or family with one presenting condition (that is, dementia) will come from two different sorts of budget, and be delivered by staff from two different sorts of system. You need to know this to make sense of some of what they will say to you. I can't give you a table that neatly sets out where you should go for occupational therapist support or tell you who provides continence support. Sometimes it comes from health, and from time to time it comes from the council, and sometimes each has a bit. Even within the NHS it varies, and occasionally it comes from the community nurses, and now and again the hospital. The NHS divides it into 'primary care' and 'secondary' services, and if you've got something exotic on a national scale it gets called 'tertiary'. And nested within any of these they might further divide the services into those provided by the older people's team or the mental health team. It's tedious, but you need to know this in case you get the wrong impression from what you are told by the staff you meet.

*The form of early-onset dementia that Alan has is quite unusual.
We live in a rural area and there was not a specialist unit nearby.
Complex and unusual cases had to travel a long way to a centre that
covered a wide geographical area. Apparently families often have to
rely on local services targeted at older people, even if the person with
dementia is younger. (Wife of Alan, 55)*

For example, you might ask about a particular service and get
the answer, 'We don't provide that.' You need to ask what 'We'
means, otherwise you might be fooled into thinking that the
NHS and social care system 'does not provide that'. What the
person is saying may be 'I, as a nurse, working in the older people's team of the secondary services based in the hospital, cannot
get that for you.' She might not mention that the council does it,
or that the community psychiatric nurse from the older people's
mental health team does it. She might not know about their services. (All of us can be forgiven for living and working in our own
little world at times.)

*I kept asking if there was respite care for younger people like Alan and
they all said no. It was the Alzheimer's Society volunteers who told me
about a centre that provides exactly this, even though you have to travel
a long way for it. Why did no one tell me this before? (Wife of Alan, 55)*

As a service user you need to remember that it is common for
a health or social care worker not to know about the whole
system. They often speak of their fragment of the system in
which you have to operate without reference to the rest, giving
you the impression that the system said, 'No.' In fact it could have
said, 'Yes. We've been expecting you. Take this, which we have
prepared for you.' Things are getting better, but while dementia
care is still a developing area, you need to remember that you
can't always trust your information source.

The management of incontinence shows the challenge. When someone stops going to the toilet in the right place it puts huge pressure on everyone. If you ask, the GP can refer you to the community continence nurse, who might manage you herself or refer you to the hospital. There is some evidence that a person with dementia is less likely to be given such a referral. You may or may not get a hospital-based continence assessment and medication, but again there is some evidence that a person with dementia is less likely to be put forward for surgery. The hospital or the continence nurse might provide you with pads and pants, or not, and social services may or may not provide a laundry service for your sheets. There is local variation on this. The continence nurse may support you wherever you live, even in a care home, or not. It is different in every area. What you will get is another example of a lottery, as if some locations win the prize and some lose. Rather than thinking of it as random and out of your control, the most productive action is to investigate really closely what is and is not available in your local area and from whom. There are organisations that can help you with information to find your way through this, but I can't tell you who they are in your local area. The most important thing I can do is to tell you that it matters what questions you ask and whom you ask.

The housing association said, 'Your aunt has to give up her tenancy and go into a home because we can't cope with her incontinence.' I asked what continence services the local health care system offers, and whether their care might remove the need for a move. They had not known enough to ask the right people. The continence nurse kept her at home for a further six months before something else happened and she had to leave. I was so grateful for that last summer of freedom and independence for her. (A.B., niece of 95-year-old woman with dementia)

What you should expect from your GP practice

The London borough had a tertiary research centre and a clear pathway of referral for younger people with a suspected dementia into the centre. This pathway was well known to local GPs, enabling patients to be seen and diagnosed quickly by the specialist team. (Margaret Perkins, LSE researcher)

Chapter 2 gives some detail of what to expect from the GP in the section on getting a diagnosis, but it all depends on where you are. One important role for the GP is to keep a register of the people with dementia in the practice. The GP has responsibility to look after both the person with dementia and the carer. That's harder if you don't share the same GP: for example, if your daughter lives in a different town. If you live in the same house and have the same doctor, the situation is more cut-and-dried. If the GP works in a health centre as part of a team that includes practice nurses, district nurses and sometimes a community psychiatric nurse, this is good as they all have something to offer. The health centre and its staff can give general health advice in the way they always have. They should help on the route to a diagnosis – they should take you seriously, do tests as described in Chapter 2 and send you forward to the memory clinic.

They should be able to give you advice on problem behaviour, such as:

- Aggression: what's causing it and what can be done to help while keeping you safe?

- Alcohol issues: is the amount of alcohol being taken too much and what can be done to help?

- Continence: is this behavioural or is there an underlying clinical problem that can be addressed, like a bladder infection?

- Depression: will medication help or is there counselling or other support?
- Driving: how and when do we get the driver's licence cancelled?
- Hallucinations: is it the dementia or the medication and what should you do about them?
- Nutrition: how do we make sure the person is getting everything they need to eat and drink?
- Sexual disinhibition: is the person being embarrassing in public or aggressive in their attentions privately?
- Skin integrity: if the person is frail or falls and gets cuts and bruises what can be done?

Help with any issues not on this list may be accessed via the GP if you are worried. Everyone is different and your GP should act as a signpost for other services. This would include:

- Referral to other health professionals, such as the podiatrist, occupational therapist, physiotherapist, counsellor, dentist, hospital consultant, optometrist, dietician, speech therapist, psychologist … any health service for specific problems.
- Advice on medication:
  - antipsychotics (also known as neuroleptics), which are fairly dangerous for some people but may be needed as a final resort;
  - antidepressants, which don't seem to work as well as other support when the person has dementia but may be worth trying as long as there are not too many other medications;
  - drug interactions, which once you get beyond four medicines start to cause problems.
- Support with assessing capacity so that powers of attorney can be set up:

- — the GP may have a form for this which confirms dementia diagnosis, and that the person is unable to understand relevant information, or retain it long enough to make a decision, weigh things up or communicate their decision.
- Direction and signposting towards carers' support and training.
- Direction and signposting towards sources of respite and social services.

What you should expect from the memory service

Memory services, sometimes called memory clinics, have different ways of operating. There is usually a team of people, including doctors. Social care professionals may also be among the staff at the local memory service. The clinic is experienced in the assessment, diagnosis and treatment of dementia. It is a good idea for the patient to take a friend or family member to the appointment. The clinic team may maintain a relationship with the patient for years, but in some cases they are handed back to the GP ('discharged') after as little as two months. The patient may get a letter from the clinic after the GP refers them, in as little as seven days, but in some places the waiting time is over six months.

In our NHS clinic there are consultant psychiatrists, geriatricians, nurse prescribers, specialist dementia nurses, occupational therapists, clinical psychologists, receptionists and administrators. We also have Alzheimer's Society dementia advisers and social care staff, but they don't work for us, just with us. We do home visits for the first assessment, but in general you'd have to come to the clinic after that unless you have a mobility problem. (Memory service manager)

The memory service will usually:

- Provide a specialist assessment to make a diagnosis or rule out dementia. It could be they suggest that you come back for re-examination in six or twelve months' time if your problems continue or get worse.

- Share the outcome of the assessment and diagnosis with you and your GP so that arrangements are put in place for your ongoing treatment, care and review.

- Offer advice to you and your carer/family about managing your condition with support from primary and community services.

- Provide advice, information and support for you and your carer, including counselling both verbally and in writing and possibly in the form of some follow-up visits from the Community Psychiatric Nurse (CPN).

- Signpost you to information, resources and facilities in primary, community and voluntary services.

A person with dementia will continue to live at home for a long time and receive health care in the same way as anyone else. It only really becomes complicated when you need extra care because of your dementia. There used to be long-stay NHS hospitals that looked after such patients. As many of them closed, the care moved into care homes, but few of those are prepared to undertake care for people who are extremely disturbing in their behaviour or extremely physically ill. A small number of NHS beds are available in psychiatry of old age units if behaviour is the issue. A lot of people with dementia when they are very ill end up in acute hospitals. In some cases the NHS will provide continuing care in the person's home or a care home.

NHS continuing care

You get assessed by NHS staff for this and, if provided, it is free. To be eligible the person (aka patient) must be assessed as having a complex medical condition and substantial and ongoing care needs. Lots of people with dementia will never be eligible for this NHS continuing care and will fall back on the local authority community care assessment (see Chapter 10). Whether the person is in a care home or their own home, they can still receive the free NHS care that everyone else gets. If they move into a nursing home (which is a different category from a care home) the NHS may contribute to the 'nursing' part of the cost. Social services or the resident will pick up the rest of the costs.

The initial assessment used in England is a checklist and then there is a full assessment if needed. You can download an information leaflet and checklist forms from www.gov.uk/government/publications/national-framework-for-nhs-continuing-healthcare-and-nhs-funded-nursing-care. Have your reading glasses and a pot of tea ready. The checklist alone runs to twenty-one pages, including guidance in quite small print. The full assessment tool is fifty-seven pages long, including sixteen pages of guidance. There is a fast-track assessment for people who are deteriorating rapidly.

Understanding the divisions

Alice was ready to leave hospital and we wanted her to come to us. She did a home visit to our house with the OT [occupational therapist] from the hospital to look at the en suite ground-floor room we had fitted out for her and we heard nothing for weeks, although we kept asking the nurses and they did not know. Eventually someone said, 'If

your mum wants to come out of hospital to stay with you she needs
to have those adaptations put in that the OT advised when they had
the home visit. Adaptations get installed by the council and we've got
no influence on how quick they can do it.' We went back home and
noticed for the first time a number of tiny paper dots on the toilet wall
that the NHS OT had stuck there. We called the council and they
claimed no knowledge. I'm infuriated because my husband is a builder
and he could have installed what was needed on the afternoon of the
visit, if only someone had said. (Daughter of Alice, 92)

It is very frustrating when you ask about something and the NHS person says, 'Oh, that's the council …' or 'We don't do that …' without advising you how to get access to what you are looking for. NHS workers are in most cases heroic, hard-working, well trained and extremely well meaning, but they sometimes explain practicalities from their own organisational point of view rather than the point of view of the patient or service user. It's improving, but you need to know how to get the best from them. The problem here has many angles. The hospital OT did not point out or explain what she was doing with the paper dots in the bathroom and what should happen next. The family did not know that the nurses aren't required to understand the social care system and so it was futile to ask them about the reason for the delay in the discharge process. The nurses did not ask the OT, who did know in good time, but when the nurses did get the answer, they and the OT only expressed helplessness about influencing the social care system.

What you need to do to navigate the complexities

• Get the diagnosis if you can as soon as you can. If the doctor is reluctant to consider that dementia might be the problem and move to a formal diagnosis, try another GP and once you have the diagnosis accept any help or visits from NHS memory clinic staff, who will be able to give you specific information about what is available.

● Keep a diary or record of the things that you want to know and tick them off as you get your answers.

● Find out from your local Alzheimer's Society, Alzheimer Scotland, Age UK or other similar organisation about whether there are groups or classes you can attend to get more information about your local NHS services. The local library often has information about resources and groups that are available. The value of these is that you will get insider information on how you can access services that the NHS may have forgotten to tell you about.

● The internet is great if you can use it. Google 'NHS dementia YouTube' and put the kettle on – there is a great deal to watch. Look at the blogs and forums on specialist websites, and there are lots of mini-tutorials on dementia. The website www.nhs. uk/Conditions/dementia-guide/Pages/about-dementia.aspx is a good place to start surfing.

In some parts of the UK, NHS post-diagnostic support workers are being appointed who can help you to navigate your local system. These workers, and other people who are experiencing dementia in their family in your neighbourhood, are a good place to start. The level and quality of service isn't the same everywhere so don't assume that this is as good as it gets for you.

What each person with dementia and their family need is different in every case, but basics include carer information and some instruction on the distinction between dementia and non-dementia problems so that you know when to seek more medical advice. In addition, advice on simple solutions for the commonest problems is really helpful, or you can give advice to your doctor now that you have this book! In an ideal world there would be continued involvement even after a person goes into a care home or nursing home from the team that knows them, but someone from the NHS should take up responsibility. The NHS ought to be able to provide nutritional and environmental advice, help your understanding of consent and capacity, and provide signposting to rich sources of guidance.

Chapter 12

The dangers of a hospital admission and how to avoid them

In the first edition of this book, Chapter 12 caused a bit of a media uproar and some anger from health professionals. To those of you who are professionals working to improve things for people with dementia and delirium, I would ask that you please don't feel insulted by the truths in this chapter. You are in the vanguard making things better, but families need to be warned that lots of places are less than perfect, and how good it is can be dependent on something as random as the person in charge on the day. Some of your work places have been transformed in recent years, but from what patients and families tell me, it's not universal.

People with dementia go into acute hospitals more often than the rest of the population, even though acute hospitals are mainly run as if every patient has perfect cognitive function. It is worth knowing how to help patients with dementia to avoid admission and what to do if your relative with dementia has to be in hospital. This is really important, because an acute hospital episode is full of avoidable dangers and can wreck stability for a person with dementia, causing chaos and distress for the rest of their life. You can be proactive to reduce these risks for your own loved ones (while others work on making hospitals safer for everyone). This chapter should help you with the ED (Emergency Department, which used to be called Accident and Emergency, or A&E), guerrilla visiting tactics, reducing the risk of pain and delirium, how to look out for medication errors and how to get out.

An acute hospital can be like a meat grinder for people with dementia – it chews them up and spits them out – so it is worth knowing how to avoid admission and what to do if your relative with dementia is in hospital.

Your local acute general hospital might be one that has really prepared itself to welcome people with dementia. It would be wise to do so, as up to 50 per cent of their patients may be either people with dementia or people with delirium, which looks similar and needs the same sort of response from staff. If this is the case, treat the rest of this chapter as of academic interest. And send me the name of your hospital, as I'd like to live near there.

The way we think about hospitals has evolved over time. What was an expensive luxury for our great-grandparents is now regarded as a routine service. A building that was once regarded with fear because so many people died there is now seen as desirable. We campaign against local hospital closures. We go there in preference to going to see our GP sometimes, as if the hospital was somehow superior and higher up the scale of effectiveness.

For people with dementia, nothing could be further from the truth. If they can stay out of hospital, so much the better. Of course, there are conditions which cannot be managed outside a hospital, but for many old people with dementia, getting admitted to hospital is the top of a slippery slope. They may have been managing perfectly well at home, but during their hospital stay things will happen that make them so unwell they never go home again. Research shows that if you have dementia you will stay in hospital longer than other people with the same clinical problem. For example, patients with dementia and a fractured hip tend not to be given as much pain relief as other patients with fractured hips. Uncontrolled pain in dementia gives rise to delirium that is often undiagnosed and untreated in hospitals. As a result, half of these patients die in six months. Since the first edition of this book, new initiatives in the NHS urge staff to 'Think Delirium' and you might even see those words on a doctor's lanyard. Awareness is improving, but it is a work in progress.

There are many examples of people with dementia going hungry and thirsty in hospital. Patients with dementia may get missed by accident at mealtimes.

When James went to hospital I tried to get in at mealtimes to feed him, but visiting out of normal times was not allowed. He kept saying he was hungry, but they dismissed this as the dementia. After a couple of days I asked why it said 'nil by mouth' above his bed, and it turned out this notice was there from the last patient and they'd forgotten to take it down. He'd not eaten for days, and they'd ignored his pleas for food. (Wife of man with dementia)

From the outside, it sometimes looks as if the person had a crisis, had to go to hospital and then it was discovered that they weren't coping. In fact, it is often just the reverse. The person who was feeding themselves adequately will for a variety of reasons not get enough to eat in hospital. The person who was managing their own hygiene will not be able to negotiate the complexities and confusion of a hospital and will start to wet themselves and be unable to stay clean. This same person who managed to be happy and live quietly at home, sleeping at night and entertaining themselves by day, will be kept awake by noise and light at night, and bored to death in the daytime, never even seeing daylight. After a few days of that they'll become noisy and irritable and may be given medication to quieten them down. It is not unusual after this to have a fall or a fracture, leading to more surgery, and a long period in hospital during which all their skills leave them as they get undiagnosed depression and delirium, which at times is ignored by hospital staff and goes untreated, leading to early death.

Delirium

Although delirium creates such a lot of problems, it is one of the least well-diagnosed and treated conditions in our hospitals. A list compiled by the president of the European Delirium Association includes about ten informal words that are used in medical notes referring to patients, such as 'knocked off', 'confused' and 'flat', which are not clinical terms but almost certainly indicate 'delirium'. In the same paper he gives some pseudo-scientific terms, such as 'acute brain failure' or 'acute confusional state', which also almost certainly suggest delirium. There is a proper treatment process for delirium and the condition is reversible, but there is no treatment for being 'confused', 'flat' or any of the other made-up descriptions. As a result of that, the patient goes untreated even though their symptoms have been described in the notes. For a person with dementia, delirium can be fatal.

When I asked the nurse how my mother was, he said, 'Confused, as usual.' I asked him what it was about her behaviour that was unexpected. He looked startled, not having expected further discussion and not realising that I teach this subject to nurses. 'She doesn't do what I ask her,' he replied. He just assumed, because she is old, that this was normal for her, rather than a temporary clinical condition that he should be working to reverse using oxygen and plenty of drinks of water, and careful reassurance. (Dementia nurse teacher)

Of course, this is a terrible human story. And it's terrible financially too. The person with dementia stays longer in hospital than others with the same condition and as a result is a greater tax burden and delays everyone else's treatment. The social services get handed back an old lady who needs a care home place, when what they had before was a semi-independent old lady who mainly looked after herself with a bit of home care. The family, if there is one, and the estate of the old lady now face the probability of having their assets stripped to pay for a situation that may have been avoidable.

People with dementia can avoid hospital in the first place by using all the advice in this book on how to live well with dementia (Chapters 6–9). Adapting the house and adopting some lifestyle changes can really make a difference. Note that the commonest reason for admission is a fall or a urinary tract infection. There is advice that will help you to reduce falls risks in Chapter 9. To be well you need a combination of diet, exposure to daylight, making enough use of light in the house, decluttering, choosing the right footwear and floor coverings, and exercise. In addition, avoiding urine infections is about making sure you drink lots of water.

In hospital, if the staff know what they are doing when they treat delirium, this ought to include:

- Hydration: the person needs to drink plenty.
- Oxygen: this is the fuel for the brain ... so extra may be needed.
- Treating the underlying cause: this may be medication or an infection.
- Reassurance: delirium is terrifying and survivors may suffer from post-traumatic stress disorder, the same psychological problem that affects people who have been in a war zone or a terrible accident, like a train crash.

Admission to hospital

Suppose you are arriving at the hospital with your elderly confused father. Here are the basics of surviving hospital for people with dementia and their carers.

First, don't leave him alone in the Emergency Department. He could be there for ages and it is worth taking time off your work to be with him. Acting now could save you money and time in the long run. It means that you can make sure he gets to the toilet or has a drink or whatever he needs to keep him well. Keep him warm if you find yourself in a draughty location like a corridor, and entertain and encourage him. At times you may also need to help him to stay cool, but remember that if he's immobile it probably feels cooler to him than to you or to the

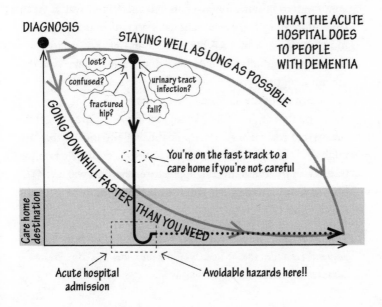

DIAGNOSIS

STAYING WELL AS LONG AS POSSIBLE

WHAT THE ACUTE
HOSPITAL DOES
TO PEOPLE
WITH DEMENTIA

lost?

confused?

urinary tract
infection?

fractured
hip?

fall?

GOING DOWNHILL FASTER THAN YOU NEED

You're on the fast track to a
care home if you're not careful

Care home destination

Acute hospital
admission

Avoidable hazards here!!

staff who are racing around. You can make sure his medication does not get missed. Hospitals are supposed to check 'cognitive status' (which means how well the patient's brain is working) on admission, but they often don't. In some cases even if they see a problem they don't take the right corrective measures anyway. If they did a careful examination they'd almost certainly know this patient has dementia or a related problem. There is a significant possibility that they won't notice it. You should tell them. You may have to mention it a number of times, because the staff member you tell sometimes does not understand the importance of what you are saying and does not write it down or communicate it. Have a notebook and a watch. At first they may say that he is not allowed to eat or drink until seen by the doctor. Pester them. Not drinking enough can make dementia much worse. Use technical words like 'dehydration' and 'delirium'. Smile.

Second, if the doctors or nurses say that they are going to admit him to hospital for 'assessment', check your watch. At the time of writing there is a national standard that says patients must not be kept in A&E for more than four hours. So if it is three hours and fifty minutes since you arrived, make sure they are not admitting your relative to hospital because they ran out of the time they are allowed to keep him at the 'front door'. Tell them you don't mind if they breach their waiting time target if it means that you can take him home today. The danger is that they might be moving him into a danger zone for a reason that is more to do with their administrative pressures than his welfare. (This is always easier to argue if you have welfare power of attorney: see Chapter 13.)

The doctor said, 'We say to relatives that we've decided to admit the patient.' He added that if he was telling the truth he'd say, 'We've admitted to decide. That four-hour window does not give us enough

time to know what we need to do, so we just bring them in, in case,
and make up our minds later.' (Relative of man with dementia)

This means that you are being admitted to hospital *in case* you've
got something wrong that needs hospital admission rather than
because the doctors *really* think you've got something that needs
it. For most of us this might be inconvenient, scary or even entertaining. If you have dementia and the admission was not really
necessary the consequences may be tragic.

Third, consider having some soft headphones and nice music
or an audiobook with you. The noise and turmoil in the waiting
area, the Emergency Department and the rest of the hospital will
make him think he has died and gone to hell. Whatever he likes
to listen to, on headphones, will reduce his stress and anxiety,
and he can shut his eyes, knowing you are there. Touch him as
much as you can, holding hands or stroking his hair. It will make
him feel better and the staff will notice. Keep yourself hydrated
and your blood sugar up, stay alert and keep good eye contact
with staff.

Fourth, don't leave your father – especially when staff ask
you to. I hear tales of carers who are sent from the cubicle when
people with dementia are examined by medics on the grounds
of confidentiality. This is silly. The person with dementia needs
someone consistent to know what is going on. Even if you don't
have a legal document, no court is going to send you to jail for
insisting on protecting a vulnerable adult. Let the doctor or
nurse carry out their examination and let your relative do all the
answering that he is going to do. If he speaks for himself and says
the wrong thing, don't interrupt. They need to hear him saying
the wrong thing or being slow, or not replying. Wait until you
are asked or until the end of the examination to point out that
he does not live where he said he lives any more, or that his age

is different from what he said, or to fill in the blanks. Also, make sure they know if he is much worse than usual. Sometimes they assume that because a patient has dementia, how confused they are at the hospital is 'baseline normal' for the patient. If it is not, make sure that clinical staff know this. If he's more confused than usual there will almost certainly be a reversible cause, and that is what the hospital needs to focus on and reverse it.

The reason for unnecessary hospital admissions of people with dementia seems to be related to hospital staff not having much experience of people with this condition, with the result that they can't believe that the person is going to survive a night at home. In addition the hospital doctor may have anxieties that if the person they are sending home has an adverse outcome subsequently, they will be held personally responsible. Interestingly, if it turns out that the hospital admission has a bad outcome that does not seem to be blamed in any way on the admitting doctor. Go home and fall = my fault. Go into hospital and fall = the system's responsibility. This is how the system makes overworked and harassed clinicians think, even when risk of an accident or adverse incident in hospital is higher. Research shows that people with dementia in hospital are more likely to have falls and other adverse incidents.

My husband was in a side room on his own and he kept trying to get out of bed. Because of his dementia he was unsteady on his feet and confused and anxious. They were worried about him being incontinent. I said, 'Please don't put a catheter in – he'll only pull it out and hurt himself. I'll stay the night with him.' But they sent me home. It wasn't allowed for me to stay. That night he did pull the catheter out and then he fell on the floor climbing over the cot sides they put on his bed to try to contain him. (Widow of 82-year-old man with dementia)

Many hospitals have brave and clever plans to overcome this perverse incentive to admit patients, including rapid-response teams and specialist nurses, but it is a serious issue that continues to cause concern. You need to keep an eye out for your relative.

It might turn out that there is something wrong that absolutely requires a hospital stay. Some hospitals are geared up for this, having a system called the 'Blue Butterfly' scheme or something similar that means staff are alerted to the presence of a person with dementia and know how to support them by discreetly identifying them with a little sign on their notes or by the bedside. They should ask you or the patient if they mind being identified in this way, as technically this would be disclosing the diagnosis to people who theoretically might not need to know. Be assured, if the patient has dementia, everyone needs to know, including domestic staff and administrators. If staff see the butterfly sign, they know what to do differently for that patient. Hydrate. Explain yourself. Repeat yourself. Keep the atmosphere calm. In fact, all the strategies covered in Chapter 8 about how to understand and manage disturbing behaviours at home should be followed in hospital.

Of course, it won't work unless staff are educated about what will make a person with dementia worse. I've seen people with dementia hurtled through a busy hospital to their destination ward on their back on a trolley by porters or other staff chatting to each other or using their mobile phones. It's a nightmare. People with dementia are incredibly stressed already, so why would health workers do something to make things worse? If your relative is in a bad hospital, you can't change that hospital, but your presence may improve or modify the behaviour of some of the staff. Sometimes it is not carelessness but ignorance of what is needed.

The GP may already have made a careful and correct

assessment that the person needs to be in hospital. Even so, the hospital is sometimes organised in a way that means they can't go straight to a bed when they get there, but have to pass through the Emergency Department and all the assessment processes as if they just came in off the street, even though the experienced GP who knows them well has already done the assessment. The patient has to bend to their systems, even though they have already been classified as fragile. Be ready to protect them.

My dad was told by the GP he was going to the hospital for assessment, but when he got there they kept asking him why he had come and what was wrong. We waited for hours for the doctors. When they arrived, they pulled the curtains round and indicated I was to go away. When I saw Dad again he had no idea what had happened or been decided and no one told me, even though I told them he had dementia and I am his carer. (Daughter of J.G.)

When a patient arrives on a hospital ward there are some procedures that ought to happen if the patient is known to have dementia, but also arrangements including specific design elements should be in place to make them comfortable.

The patient with dementia should be nursed in a single room if possible to minimise noise and disturbance. People with dementia find it hard to make sense of what they are hearing, so background noise is a greater problem for them than other people. It gets in the way of understanding what people are saying to them, or concentrating on essential tasks like eating. The chaos that can be caused by a person with dementia can agitate everyone else and set other patients off into angry or disturbing behaviour, so you can help staff understand that a single side room is not a privilege for your mum or dad, but offers advantages for their fellow patients. The controlled environment will make it less likely that his or her behaviour will become disturbing, particularly as family and friends will find it easier to stay and keep them calm. It will also be easier to keep the place quiet and dark at night, helping them to sleep. If the curtains don't fit the window, that's going to be a problem for any patient who is accustomed to sleeping in the dark. A window in the door is particularly unhelpful. The patient then sees confusing moving images in the night and will be inclined to get out of bed to investigate. Nurses say they like it for observation, but if a visual inspection was important they could prop the door open. You can't change the design, but if you are aware of the common misperceptions that people with dementia get, you can help explain his behaviour to the staff and that might prevent some inappropriate staff responses.

The ward sister said to me, 'We can't make a fuss of her just because you say she's got dementia. I've got everyone else to think about.'
I was so disheartened that I could not argue. I wanted to tell her that I WAS thinking about everyone else. Mum's behaviour is so embarrassing. You hear the other patients complaining to their visitors. But when she got moved to a side room it was much easier for her and everyone else, and I was able to stay overnight with her.
(Daughter of Ethel, 90)

The room should have an en suite toilet because getting to and from the toilet is fraught with hazards for people with dementia. In a strange environment they can't remember what they've been told about where the toilet is. Having your own is ideal, in particular if the door is open and there is good signage. Experts talk about 'architectural incontinence'. That's when the person wets themselves because the building was designed in such a way that they could not find the loo in time. All the elements that were described in Chapter 9 would help. There is a limit to what you can do to improve the design of the room for the short time you are there, but if you are aware of the limitations of the design you can work with them.

The room needs to be well lit in the daytime. There should be a window that at least shows what time of day it is by allowing daylight in, and some vegetation or a view outside makes a real difference. Exposure to daylight affects the body clock even more in old people with dementia, so it would be brilliant if there was access to an outside garden or terrace in daylight hours, especially the morning.

Our hospital has a lovely courtyard garden that you can see through the windows, but the doors are locked and no one can walk in there. (Hospital manager)

From the bed there should be a visible clock, and a calendar would be nice. If there is a metal flip-top bin the lid should be fitted with a dampener, to stop it clanging every time a doctor washes her hands and throws in a paper towel. It is possible to be prescriptive about these things in a hospital, because statistics show that every hospital room is going to have a person with dementia or cognitive impairment in it at some point. Up to 50 per cent of patients are affected. In the section of this book on home design modifications the advice is less prescriptive, because you don't want to change too many familiar elements at home. In a hospital it is inexcusable to fail to provide evidence-based dementia-friendly design and fittings. There is a limit to how much you can modify a room when it has been allocated, but if it does not have the right design features, be sure to complain to the hospital afterwards, in writing. Recommend to them the free dementia-friendly hospital design guidance that is available on the internet (dementia.stir.ac.uk/ design/virtual-environments/virtual-hospital) and point out that many of the changes are low-cost and will pay for themselves in a very short time, by the reduction of adverse incidents, like falls.

Hospital floor surfaces are often shiny and reflective. Because this makes them look wet, and people with dementia may have problems with depth perception and visual impairment, they'll be uncertain about walking on those potentially icy or slippery surfaces and might fall over as a result. It is really helpful if the environment is uncluttered. Hospitals have too many pointless signs and out-of-date notices and not enough attention is paid to essential information and way-finding needs. Bathrooms are frequently stark in their decoration, but also used as an equipment park and location for extra boxes of stores. A person with dementia being taken for a bath there would be justified in wondering what was happening if asked to undress in that situation. If your relative starts to show disturbing behaviour in this environment, you can point out the problems to the staff.

My mother does not like showers and she hated having her bath in hospital and so I went in and did it myself. We had fun, and it was relaxing for her. But I had to drape some sheets over the junk in the room to make it more homely for her. (Daughter of Keesha, 83)

Often staff will inform patients about the nurse call system. Ideally this should be a silent one involving vibrating pagers, so that the patient does not have to listen to buzzers going off all day and night or put up with flashing lights. These have been available for some time, but they are still rare for no other reason than that staff don't ask for them and maintenance departments haven't been persuaded to fit them. Of course, if you've got dementia you won't remember what the nurse said, so you won't remember how to call. Movement sensors are easily available but not often used for patients who have dementia. Hospitals do not fold round you when you have this sort of vulnerability.

Your relative should have access to plentiful supplies of fluids, unless he is on some special regimen that limits them. Be aware that the drinking jug is sometimes accidentally or carelessly placed out of reach by staff, and if it is clear plastic filled with clear water, and out of the line of sight, it might also be effectively invisible. People with dementia follow visual cues more than some others. Squirt some orange in it? Put it nearer?

General issues about medication safety

Keep a close eye on the medication. Sometimes doctors need to take the patient off previous medication to see if that is what has been making them ill. But sometimes this is not well enough thought through. For example, the person with dementia might be used to managing their own medication and they might not comply with what is going on because they are not given an explanation at every medicine round and they forget or can't work out what is happening.

When I went to see Mum in hospital she said, 'Can I come home?' and I said, 'Not till they make you better, Mum,' and she said, 'How're they going to do that, darling?' and I said, 'They'll most likely give you pills, Mum,' and she said, 'What? Like these?' And she took half a dozen assorted capsules out of her dressing-gown pocket. She said, 'They've given me the wrong ones, so I've not been taking them, and I didn't like to say they were wrong in case the nurse got into trouble.'
(Daughter of Dominka, 75)

Being given the wrong medicine is a common hazard of being in hospital. In this case it was the right medicine but the patient was trying to protect herself against being poisoned accidentally. She had dementia but she was not stupid.

Your reports of what your relative was like previously are really important. Because they are old, staff sometimes make assumptions and have low expectations for the patient, assuming they are headed for a care home. Issues that have arisen for the first time in this patient are not questioned. The assumption is that all old people or people with dementia are like this.

The painkillers that my mum has been taking have horrible side effects, we know, but when she got to hospital they took her right off them. The next day they said, 'Of course, she's incontinent, and she's had a fall ...' and I was so surprised because she never had been incontinent and they had accepted it as normal for her. I realised she suddenly got incontinent because the uncontrolled pain meant she could not move fast enough to get to their toilet and had an accident on the way. She was so upset and ended up wetting on the floor and slipping in it. (Daughter of Temeeka, 73)

A second issue is that the person with dementia is frequently started on antipsychotic medication in hospital to keep them quiet. This is the term for a range of drugs that will sedate the person when they are noisy and disruptive. Depending on what sort of dementia the person has this medication could finish them off (see Chapter 2). All medicine involves risk, and it might be that the person has to have antipsychotics as a last resort for some horribly severe and complex symptoms, but make sure that the doctors really are using them as a last resort and not just reaching for the first response they think of. Professor Sube Banerjee has reported that 180,000 old people are given antipsychotic medication every year, but less than a quarter of them get any real benefit, and about 1,800 old people die each year as a result of this particular medicine. If it was children dying there would be a riot. Our press is less sensitive to the death of older people, reflecting the values of our society. Just don't let it be your parent.

It is best practice for a hospital to start to plan the discharge of the patient the moment they arrive. The aim should be to return them home (or to their care home, if that is where they came from) with their medical problem resolved. There is evidence that hospital staff sometimes see an old person with dementia arriving from their own home, ill and dishevelled, and assume from the start that they are only ever going to be fit for a care home. The outcome for the old person is determined and fixed by this assumption. To be fair, the tendency to delay discussion about 'what next?' and 'what if?' is endemic in families as well. How many of us have had the conversation with our own children about what we want to happen when we become frail, or if we lose capacity to make decisions? Do we want to be resuscitated and treated assertively? Do we mind going into a home? How much risk are we prepared to tolerate?

It is never too soon after an admission to hospital to start the family conversation about where the person will go. Unfortunately, many people with dementia languish in a hospital for three or more months after they are able to move on, simply because we have not got ourselves into gear from the start and planned what was going to happen next. The day to check out home care services is the day the person is admitted to hospital, not the day they are described as ready to go. It is even better if you thought about it last year.

Visiting

One day I was headed towards the door of a ward to give advice about a person with dementia who was creating difficulties for the staff only to be met by an irritated nurse who all but put the palm of her hand in my face and barked, 'No visitors till three.' Disconcerted, and in fact not quite sure if I'd heard right, I stepped back.

Behind me was an elderly man with a flat cap and a small suitcase on his lap, sitting on a bench. He shook his head. 'You'll not get in till three, dearie,' he said. Glancing at my watch, I saw it was four minutes to three. So I sat beside him, even though I was meant to be working. He was desperate to get in. His wife of sixty years was in there in a terrible old nightdress that she was ashamed of and he had her nicest clothes in the bag. He'd been sitting for about half an hour, having arrived in good time with the clothes in the mistaken understanding that he'd be able to get them to her before visiting started. Dead on three the ward doors opened with a crash and the anxious relatives from the waiting area went through to make the best of the strictly limited access to their loved ones. It's not good. Staff were embarrassed about the hand in my face when they worked out who I was, but were clearly unconcerned about the personal issues for the lady or her husband. (Hospital visitor)

Open visiting for people with dementia has now been introduced in a number of hospitals, but even there the impression given is that people have to work round the system, rather than the system working for the people. There is nothing you can be doing in hospital that cannot be interrupted by staff. When I was a ward sister I had to defend an elderly patient one day when the doctor arrived, wishing to undertake an examination which involved inserting a gloved finger in his bottom. The doctor had forgotten to do that part of the examination earlier and the gentleman was now sitting up eating his dinner. As it was not a life and death issue, I asked the doctor to return later, which was clearly not convenient for her. To be honest, we argued, and it got bitter, but in the end she agreed.

It is as if there is a perverse hierarchy of need. We need to keep the system working, then we need to satisfy the requirements of staff to undertake their ritualistic tasks, then we need to address routine issues and only then the 'ordinary' things, like

sleeping, eating, having your loved ones beside you comforting
and caring for you ... These ordinary things seem so far down the
line and unimportant to staff that they sometimes get excluded.
You must work to reverse that order for your relative.

As it happens, those are the things that make most difference
to a person with dementia. Your dad is more likely to cooperate
with the staff if you are with him offering reassurance. If they
don't have time to wait for him to do slowly what you know
he can do for himself, you may be able to take that off them
and let them rush about helping other patients. The point is that
they avoid doing very much to patients during a visiting hour.
At the one time of day when they let you in to visit, they usually
don't create any opportunities for you to do useful activities like
helping with changing clothes or with eating. They treat visiting
time like my granny treated unfamiliar or posh visitors to her
house. Tidy up, stop doing anything and give a good impression.
Family visits should involve sprawling about and having treats
and laughter. No impression is needed apart from love and fun
and the eating of Jaffa Cakes. That is the sort of hospital visiting
that would be perfect for a person with dementia.

Of course, there are limits, and it depends what's wrong with
the person. But don't just sit there politely eyeing the grapes.
Do something. My advice is, be a guerrilla visitor. Find ways of
having open visiting if only for this patient. Challenge and defy
the visiting times and rules. Make rotas with friends and family
to make sure the person is not left to the mercy of the system.

Useful things to do while visiting:

- If possible, take the person with dementia for some exercise.
  It is one of the most important elements of dementia care
  (see Chapter 6). Very many people have their mobility vastly
  reduced as a result of a hospital stay.

- If possible, get them into daylight. This may mean commandeering a wheelchair, because although many hospitals have gardens, many are not easy to get to. You may have to insist on a key for access.

- Take as many personal objects – for example, cards from grandchildren, drawn pictures, photos, pot plants – as you think you can reasonably get away with and festoon their bed space. Patients who appear to have a large and interested family seem to get more attention, and objects demonstrate that. It's not a research-based observation but one can imagine why it is the case.

- Have a memory book or communications passport. This is often a scrapbook or notebook (you can get printed versions of booklets from the Royal College of Nursing or the Alzheimer's Society called 'This is Me') that allows you to record the person's likes and dislikes so there is no excuse for staff 'not knowing' when you aren't there. Don't give the staff the only copy, because they will lose it.

- Encourage eating and drinking. You need to check about any medical issues, but often there's no limit to what you can bring and they might well not be eating the hospital food. Find out what their heart's desire is. Ice cream? Belgian chocolate? Steak? Tripe à la mode de Caen? Then get it to them by hook or by crook.

- Check their ankles for swelling. If I had a pound for every old lady I find in hospital with swollen ankles, sitting up all day in a chair with her legs dangling, I'd be rich. Draw it to the attention of the staff and make sure they've got ways of keeping their feet up.

- Check their bony bits (and bum … you only need to ask) for redness and soreness. A person who does not move about enough, who is constipated and dehydrated and sometimes incontinent will get sore where the skin and bone are pressed together on their bottom or their heels and elbows. After the redness, the skin can break and become infected and this necrosis is called a pressure sore. Shamefully, they occur in people who are being 'cared for' in hospital.

- Take them to the toilet and wash their hands.

- Insist on speaking to staff about their condition. If you have power of attorney (see Chapter 13) you can do quite a lot. Nursing staff may say that you need to talk to the doctor, who is not available, and that you will need to make an appointment. That's not good enough. Insist on reading the notes. That often results in a doctor being found.

- Find a way of letting the staff know 'who' is in the bed. Did this little man in the bed once blow up some tanks? Did he bake amazing bread? Does he have twenty-five grandchildren, one of whom is a sharp lawyer who specialises in medical negligence? (I once discovered a formerly terrifying matron languishing in a hospital bed and the nursing staff did not even know that this old lady had ever been a nurse, far less that she designed most of the training they'd had.)

Increasingly, we are trying to get hospital staff to see family and friends as extra pairs of hands. If they can visit at mealtimes and help to encourage the person to eat, and eat alongside them, that's good. If they can help by making sure the patient washes their hands before eating and after, and taking them to the toilet and helping with hygiene in the way they would at home, that is great …

Bed moves can be fatal

Hospitals are under pressure to look after lots of patients as quickly as possible, because doing it slowly costs more money and there are always people having to wait in line for treatment or having procedures cancelled.

The design of most hospitals makes all of this even more difficult than it needs to be. Patients are often grouped in a 'bay' of four or six people. If they were all in single rooms it would be simple. When one patient has died in a single room or moved, another could take his place. Because the majority of patients are in a bay, if one of the ladies dies or leaves, they need another female to take up the place. If the next patient in line waiting in A&E is a male – your dad, for example – it presents a practical problem. He can't go in with five ladies. He has to have a side room, because the only available bay space is 'female'. That's nice for him. But the lady who was in that side room has to be moved to the female bay to give him his space, and that can be very confusing for her if she has dementia. A day later, after he has settled in, they might need a man to make up a space in a male bay and release a side room for a lady … so out he goes. Dementia or not, he gets moved, even though there is research that shows it is very bad for people with dementia to move. Sometimes shuffling the spaces means that the patient has to go to another ward. For example, if the gynaecology ward, which deals with specific female problems where the ladies are mainly having surgery, has a vacant female bed, an old lady might get put there to make space for a man in the medical ward. These moves can take place at any time of day or night. Just imagine how it feels to wake from a drugged sleep and find yourself hurtling again along dimly lit hospital corridors, among strangers. It is a total pain if you've just worked out where the toilet is and now you've got to work all that stuff out again in a new ward.

You go to the bed where your mum was at the last visiting time and the curtains are round a body covered in a sheet and people are talking in hushed whispers. Actually she's not dead, but the person who got her space is. She's on the terrace having a cup of tea. Not very funny. Or you arrive when the empty bed is being washed for the next person and the staff can't actually tell you very quickly where your mum is. And they say things like, 'She's gone,' and your heart stops because she is a notorious wanderer and you think they've let her leave without telling you. And the ward clerk ruffling through the records laughs and says, 'Oh, I've lost her … Where's she gone? … I've just come back from holiday and I can't find anything …'

You might not think there's much you can do about the bed-move problem. It really does not help to get angry, because the nurses in front of you feel they have little control over the system. You can manage the situation and do what you can to make sure that, if anyone is disadvantaged, it's not your loved one. Other people are responsible for the system; you are only responsible for this one person. The fundamental plan is to make sure that they only move your person as a last resort, on the understanding that you will make a significant issue about it.

First, make sure that the hospital and ward have your contact details which work twenty-four hours a day. Don't give a landline number, because if you don't answer at any time, they sometimes don't have a plan B for getting in touch with you.

I got to the hospital and Dad was dead. It was such a shock. It took me two hours to get there, and he had been dead for two hours. They said they called my home number and I had just left so they did not leave a message. My husband, who was in the house, could have called me on the mobile. The nurses could have called me on the mobile. But in those days they had a policy of not calling mobiles. I was too distressed to

drive and it took my husband hours to come to get to me to take me
home. I sat and cried in the entrance. (Daughter of Jonathan, 79)

Second, make a special request to the staff that if there is any question of patients being moved, your dad should be a priority for staying put, particularly if he is lucky enough to be in a single room. Remind them that if he had an infectious disease they'd not move him out of isolation and that dementia is like an infectious disease. For example, if he is noisy at night in a bay of patients, no one else is going to get any sleep and other relatives will complain, apart from the effect it will have on staff and patients. His dementia would affect the well-being and recovery of others, and this could be prevented by keeping him in the side room. Specifically, ask them if they could mention this to the 'bed manager'. The bed manager is an overarching nurse who has the power to tell the staff in any ward to vacate beds or move the occupant to a different place – or to leave them where they are.

Third, if a bed move happens step up your visiting and mention that you will consider making a formal complaint if it happens again, as you are aware that multiple moves pose an avoidable risk for people with dementia. You may wish to say that the only acceptable move would be into a single room, if they are not already in one.

Pain relief

There is research showing that when people with dementia in hospital are suffering pain they are less likely than other patients to be given something to help. The way you get medicines in hospitals is usually like this. First, they throw away all the pills that you've been on, prescribed by previous consultants and your

GP. Then the hospital doctor examines you and writes a prescription for use during your admission. It's often on a big chart kept at the end of the bed. This might include any of the medicines that all the previous experts said you needed. With luck the hospital doctor will have stopped only those pills that were working against each other or not working at all. Very many older people are on five or more different tablets and it is highly likely that these are making the person more ill in some way. One problem is that if the hospital doctor prescribes something which is exactly what the person was taking at home, the hospital pharmacy may issue a different tablet from a different manufacturer, so the colour or size looks different. It can be very confusing. The nurses are supposed to explain, but in practice I see little medicine pots of pills being popped down beside the breakfast tray. Leaving medicines with patients is often said to be a result of nurses being 'too busy'. Of course everyone is very busy, but this just offers opportunities for patients to put pills in their dressing-gown pocket or for other patients to inadvertently swallow them. And it is strictly against all nursing codes of practice. What does it say if hospital nurses are too busy to give patients the medicines that are meant to make them better?

The tablets, injections or intravenous drips that the hospital doctor prescribes can be given in two ways. The first is to administer the medication at regular intervals – for example, four times a day or twice a day. Sometimes the timing between pills is so important that the nurses will wake you up to give them to you. Sometimes the timing of medication can be more relaxed, and it is given at roughly breakfast, lunch, teatime and bedtime. And when the staff are busy it might be astonishingly early or late. Sometimes they just forget. The second way is that the medication is given on demand. Doctors write permission for this on the prescription chart using the letters 'PRN' or the words 'as required', only stating a limit to the number of doses. For example, you might be 'written up' for paracetamol 'for pain PRN up to four times a day'. In those cases, the nurse will come to you at the time she's giving out the other pills and say, 'Have you got pain?' and if you say yes, she'll give you paracetamol for it. If you say no, she'll perhaps ask you another time. Or you might get some in between medicine rounds if you actually complain of pain. Or not ever.

This is where the provision of pain relief to people with dementia in hospital falls down. If an old lady thinks she is at the golf club and someone in uniform looms up and asks such an odd question, she'll say, 'No', wondering why the 'waitress' has asked her this. Even if she was in pain she'd not tell them. Why should she? Often people with dementia say no at first to most suggestions. It is the safest answer if you are not sure what is going on and what they are going to do to you. This may explain why, in hip fracture cases, research shows that people with dementia get less post-operative pain relief than other patients of the same age with the same condition. In addition, many older people have some painful condition or other, like arthritis, which may get worse or feel worse in the unfamiliar routine and confines of hospital. Older people with dementia may be poor at communicating that they are in pain when asked, and may not understand the system that requires them to ask for pain relief between drug rounds. It is better practice just to give routine painkillers on a regular basis, or to give them a 'pain patch', which looks like a sticking plaster and is a transdermal preparation that slowly releases pain-relieving medicine through the skin over time.

If pain relief was a bad thing, frugality with the drugs would be a good thing. However, research shows that if a person with dementia suffers pain, they are very likely to get delirium. Delirium can be fatal, in addition to being deeply unpleasant. Rather than saying that they are in pain, people with dementia communicate their untreated pain by becoming agitated, or aggressive, or trying to leave the area. When I am consulted about disturbing behaviour in older people with dementia in hospital, my first question is routine pain relief. Sadly, many hospital workers might first reach for a sedative, like the dreaded antipsychotic medication, thus leaving the person with dementia still in pain but stupefied and wobbly on their feet.

I made the mistake of only asking, 'Is my mother on any painkillers?' because she was so agitated, and they said, 'Oh, yes!' and rattled off the names from the prescription chart. I was at the front door when I had another thought and went back up to the ward and asked a second question. 'When did my mother last have a painkiller?' and the same nurse looked at the chart and said briskly, 'She's not had any for six days.' I had originally asked the wrong question. Who knew? When she was given some pain relief she started to calm down within thirty minutes. (Daughter of Alice, 96)

It is reasonable for you as a carer to ask the ward staff what 'pain scale' they use to assess whether a patient with dementia is in pain, and ask to see the results for your relative. A pain scale is a formal method of estimating how much a patient is in pain. It might include a diagram of a body so the patient can point to where it hurts. It may include a series of questions to help decide how much pain the person is suffering. You may have heard medics on TV in emergency programmes saying, 'On a scale of one to ten, how bad is the pain in your chest?' and the patient gasps out a number. Because people with dementia have communication difficulties and sometimes can't answer a question as clearly as that, there are special pain scales that are used in best practice to decide whether people with dementia are suffering pain and where it is, often using facial expression and movement as a guide. There is extensive research on pain in dementia patients and guidance available for staff on how to assess pain. Some painkillers that work well for most of us may cause problems for older people with dementia because when they are broken down by the liver they create substances that make delirium or other symptoms worse. It's a problem. They either don't give you pain relief or they dose you with something that is going to be bad for you. Guidance on how to do good pain control is available from professional organisations and you can check whether staff are adhering to the guidance by asking, for example, if they are using one of the recognised dementia pain scales (a famous one is the 'Abbey' pain scale). Ask to see what they are using.

The main danger to look out for is your relative being given sedation to stop them expressing their pain. To be bewildered and in agony is a nightmare.

Something to do

There is a further dilemma here. If acute hospitals were working properly people with dementia who don't need hospital care would not be sitting in them for three months after they are ready to leave. On the other hand, because these waits are a reality, acute hospitals need to be providing an environment and stimulation that will help to maintain the person with dementia. It is quite reasonable to ask if you can bring the pet dog up to visit, even if the reunion has to take place in the hospital garden. You are justified in challenging the nursing staff if there is meaningless endless TV on which no one is watching. Jolly music is all very well, but no one wants it all the time (apart from some staff). Sometimes the hospital is happy for you to take their patient out for a trip home or for lunch, for example. Ask about a 'day pass', which is a formal agreement for you to take the patient away with a guarantee that the bed will be there when you get back. After all, if they have said she's ready for home, they can't detain your mum. Watch out for a tendency to overemphasise what she can't do, which would make her nervous about coming out and about with you, and make you nervous too. She might be their patient, but she's also your mum and a free citizen.

The simplest things can make a difference. Staff might arrange some chairs around a table so patients can sit in companionable silence looking at the paper and drinking tea, or they could begin to chat or start a game of poker ... anything to relieve the boredom. Nurses often require everyone to be neat and tidy beside their bed, too far away from anyone else to talk, even in the bay with five other humans. You can help to make the place more sociable. If the hospital has volunteers or a chaplain, find them and let them know that your relative would welcome a visit. Make a donation to them in cash or kind. Buy attention, if you can afford to. Ask if you can pay for a visiting hairdresser to fix their hair or beautician to come and do a manicure. Give your dad a hot shave. Don't be afraid to take some control of the environment.

There were three daughters who used to take their mother for a bath at visiting time on our ward. She loved those visits, and came out all relaxed, cleaned and moisturised and ready for bed. In anticipation I used to clean the bathroom, and one day was just leaving it when they came in. Her daughter assured me that I did not need to because they brought their own cleaning materials and toiletries and cleaned our bathroom before and after bathing her. They had actually been put off by the poor level of the hospital's hygiene and were embarrassed to say it, so they were quietly protecting their mother, and replacing what would have been a staff chore with an act of well-organised tenderness. (Jane, 59)

The use of restraint

Make no mistake, relatives are the last people to create unnecessary fuss about the use of protective restraint. On the contrary, they are afraid that hospitals will fail to protect the person with dementia. There are practical reasons why one might restrain your mother during an admission to hospital. For example, she might be trying to get outside in her pyjamas, or trying to get into a man's bed in the next ward. General hospital patients here are not usually legally detained, and being restrained under those circumstances is a serious and potentially illegal deprivation of liberty. If they take a risk and restrain someone, and no harm is done and no one complains, it might go unremarked. However, the proper use of restraint requires them to involve families or others in discussion about its use, and it needs to be reviewed.

The problem appears to be the extent to which staff fail to assess the underlying reason for the behaviour that is disturbing them. Research has been done on wandering that makes it clear that this walking behaviour is rational and not aimless. The person needs to walk about to try to clear their head, or check where they are, or relieve muscle stiffness, or get rid of tension. The worst thing you can do is try to restrict them to a chair. This sometimes gives rise to frustration, anger and aggression, which may be followed by sedation, with all the problems that are associated with it, such as falls, disturbed sleep patterns and sometimes death.

Cot rails at the sides of beds are a particular problem. They are great if your bed is being moved rapidly and you might fall out. They are very bad if you are a person with dementia.

When I was in hospital there was a confused man in our bay. He kept getting out of bed and the nurses wanted him to stay there. The care assistant was in the bay at one point when he was about to get out. She put up the cot rails on either side of the bed and told him to stay put in no uncertain terms. After she'd gone he started shuffling to the end of the bed, determined to leave. The other blokes in the other beds started shouting at him to lie down. Can you believe it? They thought they were helping the nurse by abusing the old fellow verbally. He kept shuffling and got his pyjama leg caught in the rail. Then he wet himself and cried. (Yalchin, 56)

In some hospitals cot rails are banned as a result of accidents where patients have managed to kill themselves when their head became trapped between the rail and the bed while trying to get out. If they climb over the top of the rail they may fall to the floor from an even greater height than if they just rolled off the bed. It is OK for you to object to a cot side. If they want your dad not to fall out of bed, they can offer a low-profile bed: that is, one that goes really low so he's only about a foot off the ground.

But physical restraint is not the only kind …

Last week I was in an NHS male hospital ward at about six in the evening and saw a room with eight or ten men all lying still in bed. Some were snoring noisily. It looked neat and peaceful to my colleague, but to me it looked like a Haloperidol party.* (Mark, hospital visitor)

If you think that restraint is being used you need to find out what the problem was and whether they have tried other solutions. Hospitals are required to record that they are doing it and why, and to review it regularly. And you need to tell them that for best practice they should have consulted you before using it. It is most often used for disturbing behaviour and alternatives to restraint

---

* Haloperidol is a frequently misused sedative for older people with dementia.

are described in Chapter 8. Check if they have tried those alternatives. The main danger is from the redoubled efforts of the person with dementia to do what they were planning before the restraint was placed upon them.

Going home

Nothing defines an experience like the end of it, and the end of a hospital stay can be awful or wonderful. The official guidance on discharge from hospital emphasises that the aim should be to get the person back to their own previous environment. When you have dementia, even something like a 'home' visit can be stressful, and you might not look very confident or competent in the short time that is allowed for a home visit.

The home visit is an important part of the decision about where a person is going after a hospital stay. It is like an exam that you have to pass before they'll let you out. You only really get one go and you can't swot for it. The examiner has a high standard that they expect you to meet, because they've never lived with anyone as chaotic as you were before your admission. You've actually been this chaotic since your wife died twenty years ago and it's done you no harm, but they don't like it. You'll need to do better than that if you want them to say you'll be safe at home.

I told them I'd take Dad home now because the occupational therapist was on holiday and the home visit was postponed again for another few weeks. The nurse told me that if we took him away without this OT [occupational therapist] test social work would refuse to provide services. That would mean no home help. He was making it up as he went along but it spooked Dad into refusing to come home with me. (Son)

And sometimes the home visit turns out to be quite traumatic in itself.

Mum was bundled into the little van that the occupational therapists use and whisked off to her flat, where they got her to try to make a cup of tea. She wasn't feeling very well and she had a different walking frame that she did not like, and in the course of it all she soiled herself. It's such a sad memory because she never went back to that flat, and she'd had such happy times there. She'd not met the OT before. We were told she'd 'failed' this assessment. (Daughter of Joan, 87)

Getting out

We caught up with some shopping that day and went to a matinee at the pictures and grabbed some tea before we got to the hospital at visiting time, only to discover that she'd gone home in the ambulance while we were out and about ... (Daughter of Alice, 79)

Sometimes your loved one will arrive home before you expected it. Don't be cross. Just be glad that they are home and prepare yourself for the fact that some of the community services might not have caught up with the hospital either. Sometimes when they are ready to come home, it takes a long time to get out of the system, which can seem worse.

Last time my mother left hospital, they got her dressed and sat at the end of the ward with her bag. Her bed was cleaned and someone else got in. Five hours she waited for her medication to be delivered from the hospital pharmacy. Five hours sitting in that chair, among all those sick people and their germs. Five hours. So this time she was coming out I took her home without the pills and went back and I sat waiting for the pills by myself. They weren't happy because they were supposed to explain them to her, but I told them I'd be doing that every ten minutes anyway, so they gave them to me and I left.

Don't get me wrong. They saved her life and I love them for that. They just don't have a clue about dementia. (Daughter of Aarika, 75)

Chapter 13

Some important legal issues

If you have dementia you will probably reach a position where you won't be able to make decisions for yourself. There are robust legal processes that you can set up in advance to make sure that this does not lead to things happening to you outside the range of what you'd find acceptable if you were on the case. You can set the controls while you are still able, and choose a person who will make proxy decisions for you if something completely unpredictable crops up. Because you know them and trust them and have spent time talking to them, you can relax and know that you'll be OK, since they know and understand what you want and can guess what you would have wanted if something unexpected happens. Getting wills and powers of attorney sorted is a smart move for any adult at any age, but when you know you have dementia, you need to move quickly on these. At some later stage the lawyer or doctor might stop listening to you because they decide you lack the capacity to make a decision in your own interest. Time to get advice!

Those who need to know about this include people with dementia, their families and friends. Some of you may be asked to act as attorneys or guardians, and you might apply to be a deputy. The law is really meant to be helpful, but that can't happen if you don't know how to use it and use it in time. These technical terms arise from the different mechanisms that are available.

Because this book is mainly about dementia, the information here is relatively sketchy, and you must always check up with the rules at the time you are reading this, not the time I am writing it. There is a useful list of contacts at the end of this book.

On my website www.juneandrews.net you will see a follow-up to this chapter written by a retired district judge, Gordon Ashton OBE with his own thoughts and experiences. He says:

If it is concluded that there is a lack of capacity to make a decision or range of decisions (the functional test) and this is due to 'an impairment of, or a disturbance in the functioning of, the mind or brain' then the statutory procedures for delegated decision-making can apply. In Scotland this requirement is replaced by the existence of a 'mental disorder'. These requirements (known as the diagnostic test) are intended to prevent delegated decisions being imposed on a person simply because they are eccentric or for some other inappropriate reason.

The legal system has a hierarchy of laws becoming more specific the closer they get to you. Human rights and European legislation has influenced all UK legislation and there are UK laws, but in addition each part of the UK – that is, England, Wales, Scotland and Northern Ireland – may have different specific legislation. Some things apply to one or two parts of the UK – for example, to England and Wales but not to Scotland or Northern Ireland.

At the early stages of dementia you still have the capacity to do everything you ever did. As time goes by your capacity is judged by how well you understand and recall information and weigh up options. It might even be that you do understand but you are unable to demonstrate that you do, as sometimes happens with a stroke. Talking about all these matters well in advance is really important.

I'm in my fifties with no sign of a stroke or dementia or anything so I'm not worried. But I have had a number of conversations with my daughter over the years, right from when she was quite young. She'd sometimes say, 'That's enough ...' and walk away, apparently bored, but in fact I've discovered she was retaining it all. Now she has hit the legal age, we've got the power of attorney sorted so, if or when something happens to me, she can take over. I've told her that if I'm in a home and don't know her any more she doesn't need to visit, but just check them out regularly to make sure they are doing the right thing. I know and love her now enough for all my life and the life to come. What might happen after dementia does not matter to me. (Fatma, 56)

A person who no longer has the capacity to understand a complex issue like managing a share portfolio or selling a house might still be capable of deciding what to wear, what to eat and where to go on holiday. So capacity is not an 'all or nothing' issue.

Advance decisions

There are different names for the process of making a statement about how you'd like to be treated in future when and if you lose the capacity to express an opinion. They are called 'living wills', 'advance statements', 'advance directives' or 'advance decisions'. In some cases there is a technical difference between these, but you will find people using them interchangeably. When you are ill and can't speak for yourself, such as after an accident, doctors and nurses have a legal obligation to act in your best interests and normally they decide that for themselves, particularly in an emergency, and ask questions later. These types of advance statements tell them that you have decided in advance that you want them not to put you through a particular process or procedure or treatment. An example is a Jehovah's Witness, who will say in advance that they must not be given a blood transfusion, even if the doctor thinks it will save their life. So who knows about the existence of your statement and where it is stored is quite important. Some ladies have it in their handbag. Some nurses never look in the bag in time. Crucial people, including your GP, knowing about and recording your wishes is useful.

England and Wales

The Mental Capacity Act 2005 provides a legal framework for advance decisions. The act has a Code of Practice giving guidance on how it works. Age UK has a fact sheet (Fact Sheet 72). It points out that 'An advance *decision* is a decision to refuse treatment; an advance *statement* is any other decision about how you would like to be treated.' Both get informally called 'living wills'. The doctor would be legally bound by your advance 'decision', but is only required to take your 'statement' into account. Queries can be addressed to the Office of the Public Guardian, based in Birmingham. Information about that office can be found at www.justice.gov.uk/contacts/opg.

There is a separate office for such queries in Wales and information can be found at wales.gov.uk/topics/health/publications/health/guidance/decisions/?lang=en.

Scotland

The Adults with Incapacity (Scotland) Act 2000 provides a similar legal framework to England and Wales. One difference is that the advance *decision* is not legally binding in the same way as in England and Wales, where it is governed by common law rather than by legislation. Arguably, it boils down to the same thing from the point of view of the patient or carer. In addition, there is a special type of advance statement about dementia or other mental illness treatments. If you've been detained in hospital and deprived of your liberty under the Mental Health Act* and/or are being treated against your will, even at home, you can state in advance that there is a particular treatment you don't want, and it is binding on the doctors. A 'named person' can intervene on your behalf. It's unusual, but an example might be a younger man with frontotemporal dementia who has really disturbing behaviour and falls foul of the law. He could end up in prison, a secure hospital or detained in a psychiatric ward. Someone needs to argue on his behalf about whether that's appropriate. The Mental Welfare Commissioner (www.mwcscot.org.uk) and the Office of the Public Guardian (www.publicguardian-scotland.gov.uk) would both have an interest.

Northern Ireland

As in Scotland, the advance *decision* is not legally binding in Northern Ireland in the same way as it is in England and Wales – it's governed by common law rather than legislation. See www.nidirect.gov.uk/index/information-and-services/pensions-and-retirement-planning/home-care-and-community/carers/guide-to-information-for-carers.htm.

What might you be thinking about?

Your advance decision might be to refuse treatment, even if that causes your death. You can't insist on treatment, only refuse treatment. The doctors are legally bound by it in England and Wales, and their insurers advise them that it's regulated by common law in Scotland and Northern Ireland and that the courts are likely to support a clear directive from the patient. So it is a good idea

---

* The Mental Health (Care and Treatment) (Scotland) Act 2003.

to discuss it with your doctor and make sure it is in your notes to have the best chance of control over what happens next, if you lose capacity. Tell the family too, in case the medics do not see this message in your notes in time and just ask the family for an opinion in the meantime. The last thing you want is for everyone to have done their best – only to say 'Oops' the next day when they discover your note, while you are vegetating in intensive care after an aggressive and relatively unsuccessful attempt to resuscitate you.

If you are trying to say in advance that you want to refuse 'life-sustaining' treatment like artificial nutrition or hydration even if your life is at risk, the decision has to be in writing and signed by you and witnessed. An example might be that you decide, if you have dementia and subsequently develop cancer, you don't want it to be treated but want to be kept comfortable and die naturally. (Interesting fact: research shows that people with dementia get less cancer than the general population.*) A more likely scenario is that a person with dementia might get pneumonia or suffer a stroke. Pneumonia used to be called 'the old man's friend'. People died of it peacefully in their sleep. Now that we can treat it intensively with antibiotics and intravenous infusions and life support, you are less likely to die from it. But you could choose in advance to say you don't want aggressive treatments. It's important to know that you can't use an advanced decision to demand assisted suicide or euthanasia, but you can ask for nature to be allowed to take its course while you are given tender loving care. In any case you should review it regularly and you can cancel it at any time.

You might decide that if the time for hard choices comes you want someone else to make that decision at that time about the

---

* See www.medscape.com/viewarticle/806944.

sorts of issues that would otherwise be captured in your advance statement, and make that person your attorney. You do this by creating a power of attorney, or enduring power of attorney. Again, the attorney takes your views into account but they are not legally bound by them. There are two sorts of attorney. One is for property and affairs, the other for personal welfare. It's the welfare one in particular who needs to know about any advance decision about life-sustaining treatment, as they will be in a position where they can tell the medical staff on your behalf if there is any debate about it.

So an advance statement can be:

- an advance *decision* that refuses specific treatments, like resuscitation from a heart attack;
- a more generalised statement that says 'no life-sustaining treatments if I've got no chance of getting better';
- a plea to 'give me everything that is available at the time';
- a statement of values, not just about clinical care and treatment but about what life means to you – for example, 'life in a dependent state when I don't know my relatives is of no value to me';
- a statement of who should be consulted (if this is a person you've given welfare power of attorney they can actually make decisions, not just be consulted).

If it all ends up in a dispute, that can go to the Court of Protection in England and Wales. The court can say if your advance decision is valid, and if it is they can't overturn it. In Scotland and Northern Ireland the situation is different and all a lawyer can do is predict what the court would say in each case.

What is mental capacity?

In all of the countries of the UK the guiding principle is that a person has the right to be assumed to have capacity to make their own decisions unless someone proves otherwise. All practicable steps have to be taken to support the person with dementia in making decisions. And they must be allowed to make eccentric or unwise decisions.

If you ask my mum anything in the afternoon she always says, 'NO!' and I'm pretty sure she has no idea what is being suggested. Yet, the next morning, and every morning, she'll enter into a sensible conversation about the same thing. (Eleanor, talking about her mother, Jane, 80)

Dementia is overwhelmingly tiring, and if you check out the person in a darkened room later in the day when they are hungry and thirsty and just waking from a nap, they won't make as much sense as they could at another time of the day. Is this not true of all of us to an extent? It's just that the rest of us are not at risk of someone overriding our decisions because they think we're not very smart. You will know when the best time of day is to give the person the best chance of thinking about what they really want.

Another principle is that if a decision is made on my behalf the person making it needs to prove that they're doing so in my best interest, and that the least restrictive decision is being made. So you might think that I can't manage my finances, but I can still have enough money for shopping for shoes you think are expensive and unsuitable. The vexed question is sometimes about who decides.

The lawyer would not let George change his will because he wasn't sure if he had the mental capacity, and she said we needed to ask the doctor. The doctor said that wasn't a clinical decision – it was a legal one. George was stuck in the middle. (Wife, 71)

Practical suggestions about money

If a bank becomes aware that an account holder has lost mental capacity it will freeze the account until an attorney or a court order fixes that. But while you still have capacity, some of the following mechanisms might make life easier:

- Set up as many direct debits and standing orders as you can so that bills get paid regularly without you having to handle them.
- Think about having a joint bank account with the person who has power of attorney. This means that they can access any of your money that is in that account, and if you trust each other, that is convenient. While you are unwell or in hospital you could say to them, 'Send a cheque for £25 from our joint account to Doris for her birthday,' and it would be done. Or you could say, 'When you are in town, will you get me out some cash from the ATM?' and they can just do that and bring it to you.
- Think about a third-party mandate. This is an instruction to your bank or building society to provide access to your account for another person. However, if you lose capacity, the mandate is terminated, so it's not that useful for dementia in the later stages.
- If you have a Post Office card account for benefit payments you can apply for another person to have their own card and PIN number so that they can have permanent access to your account and withdraw up to £600 per day.

- If you can't get out to the post office the Department for Work and Pensions will make payment by cheque, which you can authorise by signing on the back and send someone else to cash for you. Get the leaflet from the British Bankers Association called 'Banking for people who lack capacity to make decisions'. There is one for England and Wales which describes helpfully three roles: an attorney, a receiver and an appointee. There is a separate guide for Scotland but as yet none for Northern Ireland. They can be found at www.bba.org.uk. There is great advice on this website: www.moneyadviceservice.org.uk/en/articles/if-the-person-you-want-to-help-has-lost-mental-capacity

In England, if you need access to the money of a person who has no attorney you will have to go to the Court of Protection. Say it was an emergency, like needing urgent plumbing work done or repairs to the central heating, someone would have to pay and then claim the money back via the Court of Protection. Even if it is the wife who wants access to the couple's joint account, the bank can freeze it if the husband has lost capacity and not created an attorney. Get one for each other on your next birthday … even if dementia is not on the horizon. It's like insurance: pay now or expect trouble later.

In England there is a power of attorney that works only when you have mental capacity. It's like getting your lawyer to make decisions for you while you are on holiday. That's not so useful for dementia. For that, in England and Wales you need a lasting power of attorney (LPA). In Scotland it is just called a power of attorney.

In each country there are two types:

- one for property and money affairs;
- one for care and welfare issues.

And in Scotland there is a third type in addition:

● one that does both of the above.

When you set them up you must pay for them to be registered at the Office of the Public Guardian – there is one for England and Wales, and one for Scotland – or the Office of Care and Protection in Northern Ireland (the addresses are given at the end of the book). You can't get a paid care worker to be an attorney. Check for current rates and rebates on the websites of these organisations (at the end of the book) but it is around £82 each in England and Wales. If you get the form wrong and need to resubmit you have to pay about half of that again each time.

We are a family of four children and our parents wanted everyone to be involved, so my brother and I are joint welfare attorneys and my older brother and sister are joint property and finance. This increases the chance of there being someone nearby who can sort problems.
We signed all the paperwork at a great lunch party at my brother's house, and my mother immediately said, 'Thank goodness for that. Now will you make me go on a cruise, please?' I said I'd love to but as the welfare powers don't kick in until she has lost capacity she has to make that decision for herself! (Daughter of Frank and Catherine, 82)

To set up a power of attorney you can:

● use a solicitor;
● get forms from the Office of the Public Guardian or the Office of Care and Protection.

Lawyers do charge fees, but in some circumstances some lawyers can be provided through legal aid. It's a personal choice to use one or not and it depends on your own confidence in these matters.

Age UK, the Alzheimer's Society and Alzheimer Scotland all have useful information on their websites. Remember that this chapter is not providing legal advice but general information and everything changes, so get the most up-to-date information from the web, the Citizens Advice Bureau, or health and social services staff, and make sure that you take account of whichever country you are in.

A more expensive and time-consuming option is to lose capacity and then find that someone who cares about you has to go to a court of law to get authority to make decisions on your behalf. If no one in your family offers, the local authority will do it.

In Scotland you have to apply to the Sheriff Court and it takes at least six months. That is a long time if your boiler has to be fixed or you need to pick a care home. It involves a hearing in the court before the sheriff, usually in chambers or closed court. The guardian if appointed has to submit an inventory of the estate and a management plan. There is another process called an intervention order for approving just one thing, like the sale of a house, but the process is similar to guardianship, so if you are likely to have to take more than one decision guardianship is more appropriate. It can be an expensive and lengthy business, and at times families fall out about it and can object in court, and the guardianship itself is subject to regular reviews.

Some useful terms

Appointee (UK)

The Department for Work and Pensions is contacted through your local office to say that you would like to collect and bank benefits on behalf of the person with dementia. After consideration they will give a letter confirming that you are the appointee.

Lasting Power of Attorney (England and Wales)

The person has completed this process when they still have the mental capacity and the Court of Protection registers the power of attorney (EPA). It is then registered with the court after mental capacity is lost and the attorney can then manage the person's affairs. Enduring powers of attorney have been replaced by lasting powers of attorney, but can still be used if they were made and signed before October 2007.

Deputy (England, Northern Ireland and Wales)

Usually a close family member or someone else who can be trusted applies to the Court of Protection to act as a deputy for the person and to manage their bank account and money. The court appoints that deputy and gives a 'receivership order'.

There are really clear instructions on these matters at www.gov.uk/power-of-attorney/contact-office-of-the-public-guardian.

Chapter 14

What to look for in a care home

Choosing a care home is one of the most expensive and emotional decisions you will ever have to make, and it is hard to know what is best and how to work out if the home is continuing to provide what is needed afterwards. There is a companion volume to this one, *Care Homes: The One-Stop Guide*, but a book on dementia needs a chapter like this one to itself. In this chapter we'll go into what a good care home looks like and the financial considerations. If you were to believe all the frightening news stories that abound, you'd naturally be pessimistic about the possibility of having a good time in a care home, or being content to let your parent or spouse go to live in one.

Far too many care homes are dumps, in every sense of the word ...
Last year six 'carers' at the Winterbourne View home in Bristol were
jailed for 'cruel, callous and degrading' abuse of elderly residents.
This awful place is unlikely to be unique. Why are we afraid of ending
our lives in care? Because far too many care homes are ... uncaring,
shabby places that are incapable of showing human compassion
when it is needed the most. (Tony Parsons, from 'Why I'd rather die
in Dignitas than live in the torture chambers of a British care home',
Mirror, 2 March 2013)

Although this case was many years ago, it still shapes thinking.

The number of people who end up in a care home is relatively small, but it varies across the UK. In general you have less than a 20 per cent chance of ending up in a care home, even if you are over seventy-five. In Northern Ireland, the number of people in care homes in the first decade of the twenty-first century was higher than anywhere else in the UK. The reason for this is not known, but it is probably that families have a positive view of care homes – more positive than Tony Parsons in any case. Also there may have been less pressure on public spending, meaning that local authorities had budgets that would allow them to make placements at levels unheard of in England. But even in Northern Ireland there are huge changes, shutting NHS care homes and increasing the pressure for care in the community.

Care homes can be privately owned, or run by the statutory health or social care services, or run by the 'third sector', which means non-profit, voluntary-sector or charity organisations. The majority of privately owned care home beds are managed by very big companies, like Barchester, Bupa or Four Seasons. Voluntary-sector ownership of homes has increased over the last thirty years. Only about one in ten homes are in council or NHS ownership and that proportion continues to fall. Newer purpose-built homes are replacing the 'mom and pop' care homes which were more common in the 1980s and 1990s. At that time property prices were rising and there was an increasing market for care home places because long-stay hospital beds were closing. This meant that a couple – for example, a nurse and her husband – might take out a mortgage on a big house and make a lot of money not only on the fees for care, but on the increase in the value of the property. The property crash and the tightening of the fees that social services were prepared to pay meant that a lot of those businesses folded. Many were unviable if their beds were not full. Improved standards in relation to sharing rooms and the availability of en suite facilities, and the more discriminating customers in the self-paying market, meant that purpose-built, larger homes were more financially viable. The better-performing homes tend to have a higher percentage of self-paying customers – people who pay for themselves rather than having the council pay for their place. They often pay more than the council is prepared to pay, so in one sense those higher-paying residents 'subsidise' the situation for the residents who are dependent on council fixed rates. In return the council-funded residents give the care home business an economy of scale that benefits the private residents and stabilises the service. Everyone wins?

The collapse of the large care home group Southern Cross in 2012 was long predicted by industry insiders. Although Southern Cross homes were paid large amounts of public and private money to look after people, they had entered into risky financial arrangements using the property prices of their premises as collateral. This meant that the care home operators were very dependent on being able to pay back their loans. If the interest rate was impossibly high, the maintenance of standards became impossible. These homes became less and less attractive to families and local authorities, who took their business elsewhere, and the bed occupancy dropped, causing a further downward spiral in the viability of the homes. Although there were some scary headlines, every one of the homes was taken over by other operators, so no elderly residents were thrown out in spite of the public anxiety. A number of the homes were closed subsequently by the companies that took them over, but in a controlled way. When old people have to move from one care-home setting to another, there is said to be an increased danger of a bad outcome for them, and the stress of a move is said to lead to illness and hastening of death. The research on this is scant, and it depends on why the person had to move and how much planning was involved.

The size of the market is vast. There are over 17,000 individual care homes in England, with almost half a million beds. The top ten providers account for over 90,000 of those beds, with Bupa and Four Seasons accounting for about 20,000 beds each. Barchester and HC One have more than half that number each. There are smaller care home groups with as many as 3,000 or 4,000 beds who often score better on the measures used by the regulators such as the Care Quality Commission in England at the time of writing, so size is not necessarily a guarantee of quality or stability. But everything can change very quickly as homes are bought and sold. When choosing a care home, the quality of the management in the actual premises that you are looking at makes the biggest difference no matter who owns the home. The picture is similar in all four countries of the UK.

What does good look like?

Phone, write to or email a number of homes and ask about the level of care provided for dementia, the fees and the waiting lists. You will be able to see recent inspection reports on the inspectors' website or ask the home to send you a copy. Visit the places that are interesting. Websites always look nice. That's what the design company is paid for.

In a good home you will experience friendly greetings, a homely and welcoming atmosphere, a clean and pleasantly decorated environment and the right smell. You will probably have a sense of what is good when you see it, as long as you are not taken in by hotel-type decor that looks elegant but is not right for dementia. The first visit is probably best done on your own or with a friend who knows about or has experience of care homes. If you think that the place is promising, you can follow up with the potential resident and see what their reaction is. Some places offer day care or respite, and that would give you a chance to test and try before you make a decision. Some people think about having a trial residential period before signing a contract. It's not clear what the benefit is of that. If it is not good, you are going to move the person even after a trial. The home is on trial for the whole period that they are caring for your loved one.

The sort of things you are looking for include:

- Is everyone treated with dignity and respect? This starts with how you are treated, but when you are visiting, how do staff members refer to residents? Do they talk about 'them' as if 'they' are not there, or do they address residents as respected clients? Do they call them by their name or some general endearment? Are people treated like adults? You would expect to see a written philosophy about this and some evidence that it is used in staff training with visible results.

My uncle was Professor John Edmund Baird. Nearly everyone called him Professor Baird. Only his wife and mother had called him anything else and that was 'Edmund'. I discovered the staff were addressing him as 'John' and 'darling' and I was concerned. In a lucid moment he told me, 'I don't want you to tell them my name is Edmund. This way I know who they are – impudent strangers.' (Anne B., niece)

- In the public areas, if there is a TV on is anyone watching it, and is the programme relevant to the residents? What are people doing in the day room, and is there a staff member with them? Are residents involved in activities, nicely dressed and groomed, alert and interested? Do residents talk to you? If not they are clearly used to being ignored. Can you see people doing things for themselves – laying tables, reading a book? Of course there may be a tired person sleeping in a chair – but not everyone.

- Do the staff and the systems focus on the abilities of the person with dementia? It is probably quicker and easier to dress and feed someone than to help them to do it for themselves. If a staff member makes the decision for them about this, is it in the interest of the resident with dementia? You need to ask them some questions about dementia and judge their answers for yourself. Not least, ask them what training they've had.

- Everyone should have a care plan that is regularly reviewed; staff should all have recognised training in care planning. A large part of that is the importance of meaningful activity. The care plan should include as much as possible of the person's life story so that their routines and relationships can be respected and maintained. Does the plan single out one worker who is the key contact for the resident, taking a particular interest and looking out for them consistently over time?

- Do staff knock and wait for more than a heartbeat for a reply before entering rooms? Dignity and privacy are not preserved if the knocking and entering are all in one swift movement. It is a good clue when staff are showing you round if they take you into a resident's room, even in their absence, without asking permission. Watch how staff talk to each other and to residents while you are there. Remember, this is when the care home providers are on their best behaviour.

- Will the resident be able to choose their food, and when they eat? What happens if they are hungry or fancy a hot drink in between mealtimes? Can you share a meal with them, or make some tea?

They showed me a sample lunch menu and I asked if there was a vegetarian option. The cook replied, 'Oh, we have that at supper time.' (J.A., home visitor)

- What opportunities are there for exercise and outdoor activities? Is the garden open access and with a dementia-friendly design, including things to do and see, places to sit, and safe walking. Are there any animals, like chickens or rabbits? You'd expect there to be an active programme of external visits, whether that is visiting a café or pub, or going somewhere interesting, like a local park or the seaside. And how is it recorded? You're not interested in how many times there is a trip to the seaside. You want to know how many times your relative will be on it.

I asked if there were any parties or events, and they described a Royal Baby party in great detail. When I asked if Esme took part they said it was a shame because she was not well that day. It almost felt deceitful and it certainly would have been misleading if I had not asked the second question. (Legal representative and attorney)

- In the bedroom is there space for personal possessions and for storage? You need a place for at least two people to sit and chat. An interesting view can be really important. I know that people are anxious about balconies, but at the Dementia Services Development Centre (www.dementia.stir.ac.uk) we like them, if they are properly designed and used.

- What is done about security? If there is a resident who tends to abscond, it is wrong to lock everyone else up. Use of assistive technology by the home is to be expected for this purpose. Are they so obsessed with security that you can't open a window and get fresh air? Air quality is really important. No one wants to live out their days in a stuffy atmosphere.

- Does the home respect cultural differences in both activities and behaviour of staff? Can people maintain relationships with the outside world and the community within which they were living before the care home?

● End of life care is a very important issue. It is never too soon to talk about what is to happen.

I was a bit shocked when Dad was moving in and they asked me what was to happen when he died. I mean, of course he was going to die, but they were asking all about funeral directors, cremation, etc. If he got ill and there was not much hope did I want him moved to a hospital, or what? When the time came and he did die I was so glad we had got all that over with. They were so comforting and helpful and it really made a very difficult experience easier for me and my mother. (H.B., son)

The building

The Dementia Services Development Centre at the University of Stirling has discovered an interesting anomaly in the design of care home buildings. Over twenty-five years of supporting dementia-friendly design, it has found that what appeals to those who are choosing a care home is not the same as what works well for people with dementia. A home designed to look like a country house hotel, with soft lighting, subtle colour schemes, gilded mirrors, and hidden and discreet toilet facilities, leading off to corridors with rows of identical hotel room doors, will often win industry prizes. However much this style appeals to families and people making decisions on behalf of others, it is not necessarily right for people with dementia, according to the research.

To help a person with dementia the ideal design is much brighter and more obvious. A big coloured toilet door just off the dining room helps avoid the problem of being 'caught short' during a meal. The effect of light on the person's capacity to work out what is going on has already been emphasised, so bright light is needed. You don't want elegant drapes and pelmets across the windows if they reduce daylight. Highly contrasting floor coverings and wall coverings are important to help with mobility and visual impairments, including problems with depth perception. This might not seem so comfortable or even luxurious at first. It's more Balamory than Balmoral. More like children's nursery decor than country house hotel. But it is also more useful.

In discussion it is often said that not everyone in a care home has dementia and so homes don't need this. The sad truth is that with the reduction in public resources for care, no one is funded to go into a care home until they are quite frail. Research is starting to show that around 90 per cent of care home residents have dementia, even in care homes that do not claim to specialise in this form of care. Where people once lived in care homes for years, a residential lifetime of eighteen months is now more likely, and many residents do not reach that milestone. The chances are that in future the care home resident in general will be frail, very elderly and have at the very least the early stages of dementia.

The dementia-friendly design concept is based on a mixture of research involving people with dementia, extrapolation from the needs of people with sensory and physical impairment, and knowledge of what the international consensus is on best practice. The dementia-friendly building is comfortable and elegant, but not in the way that people might think if they have a Victorian coaching inn in mind. The person is unlikely only to have dementia and may also have other illnesses and impairments that come with great age. There are care homes which are focused on the needs of a particular social group or cultural community, such as military veterans' homes, or care homes for Jewish or Polish people. They may have design features that reflect the history and culture of the residents in general. However, because the home is only ever going to be 'home' to any individual for a short time, it has to follow certain general rules, while offering the maximum flexibility in the person's own space. If it has to be homogeneous and work for a lot of different people, let it at least be based on research evidence about what works, and not this season's palette from the interior design catalogue.

Architecture and design prizes are given for a range of reasons that may not be related to dementia design principles. If you want to compare the home you are seeing with a high standard, there are examples of ideal room layouts at dementia. stir.ac.uk/virtualhome.

Homes should offer a domestic-like environment. This means that if it is quite large, it should be broken down into smaller units. En suite facilities are required for all new and newly registered buildings. People should only share a room by choice and no more than two people at a time. If two are sharing they should have another room for their personal use – as it were, a bedroom and a living room. All the design features highlighted in Chapter 9 work for care home settings. The judicious use of assistive technology means that even if you have lost your own home, you can still have the privacy of your own space.

Staff

There may be no government standards for the level of dementia training for staff but very many care homes do have standards. Particularly in the independent sector, managers are aware that staff dementia training has three distinct and money-saving advantages. First, it reduces staff turnover by improving staff morale, and staff turnover is rather expensive. Second, it reduces adverse incidents, which are damaging both financially and for reputational reasons, because old people get hurt and the complaints and aftermath are time-consuming. And third, it improves standards of care, which is good for business, because good care homes are at a premium and filling those beds is what keeps the business healthy. So even if they have a heart of stone, enlightened self-interest makes operators inclined to take advantage of some of the low-cost and free dementia education that is available. Large care home groups often have in-house trainers.

Ask what education people have had. It is more impressive if the training is from a reputable provider such as a university, or if it is accredited by an external organisation like City and Guilds or the Royal College of Nursing. Online degrees are useful for imparting knowledge but don't always automatically change practice. Don't be over-impressed by computerised courses for frontline staff. The most important element in improving care is the face-to-face teaching that imparts moral standards and personal values, in addition to the practical hands-on skills that are vital for the job. Staff learn how to talk to people with dementia from their leaders, who set the tone and standards for the place. It is really important that someone on the team has a formal dementia qualification. There was a time when such qualifications were rare, and just being kind and doing your best were better than nothing. That's history. Staff need to have national vocational qualifications that are set down from time to time by the inspectorate. However, they also need to know about dementia, which is not a regulatory requirement. You need to ask.

The core staff of a good home must include people with responsibility for social and recreational activity, cooks, grounds staff, housekeeping staff, drivers and administrators, and all of these should have dementia training as well. In addition to the core staff you would expect some or all of the following (and maybe others too) to be available at regular intervals and on call as required:

- barber, hairdresser and/or beautician;
- dementia liaison nurse or community psychiatric nurse;
- dentist;
- faith leaders for all faiths – chaplain, priest, rabbi, pastor, imam, preacher, minister;
- general practitioner;
- librarian or mobile library;
- local befrienders;
- masseur and/or exercise leader;
- musician and/or art therapist;
- occupational therapist, physiotherapist and/or dietician;
- optometrist;
- pet therapist;
- podiatrist;
- psychiatrist of old age;
- social worker.

My favourite care home has a twice-weekly visit from the ice-cream van, complete with chimes. So I'd put that on the list as well.

Funding

Funding of care, whether in a person's own home or a residential or nursing home, is complicated. Getting information can be difficult and the rules can be hard to understand. In the past they were applied differently in different parts of the country. The process of applying is time-consuming and often bewildering. (Alzheimer's Society)

The system of payment for care homes is often seen as unfair, because people who worked and saved have to pay and people with no resources get support. Staying in a nursing home will cost almost £45,000 a year at 2018 prices on average, with the actual cost depending on geographical location as much as other factors. Thinking about how you are going to fund this in future is crucial, and you can assume prices will not fall. Care homes that provide nursing care are generally more expensive than care homes that provide residential care. The latest information on benefits needs to be sought, along with information about the person's current financial position, in order to work out what you are able to do. There are useful organisations that can help, in addition to the support that's available from social workers. When looking at information on the internet, be sure that it applies to where you are living, as each of the four UK countries has a different system, and within England local authorities differ from each other.

In general, if you've got more than between £23,000 and £24,000 in assets you will have to fund all or part of your care. If you've got less money you may still have to make a contribution. You need to check these numbers at the time. When your wealth is calculated it includes the savings and investments that you have and also the value of your house, unless the house is occupied by your spouse, a relative over sixty, a disabled relative or a child under sixteen.

It's not possible to say how long you will stay in a care home. The average length of stay has been dropping, not least because people can't afford it for long and even local authorities can't afford care home places as easily as they used to. If you are relying on savings, you need to be sure that you've got enough to last your lifetime. You could sell your home and buy an annuity. That's a financial product where you pay a lump sum to an insurance company. They are betting that you die before you've had all the money back. You would then have paid more than you needed, but at least you would never have had to worry about the money running out. An equity-release scheme lets you borrow money on the value of your house. That money could theoretically run out.

It is not known how many people have sold their homes to pay for care. The idea of older people 'having to' sell their houses to pay for care is highly controversial and successive governments have struggled to find a politically acceptable and affordable solution. In 2019 a House of Lords debate made it clear that the problem with social care in England is lack of funding.

If you are reliant on the local authority, it will decide both whether a care home is needed and what funding assistance will be given, as was described in Chapter 10. You or your family can 'top up' what they are prepared to spend in some circumstances. This means you can upgrade the services by having the council pay for the basic package, and then pay extra for something more, like a bigger room or a better view. Even if you pay your own fees, you may be able to claim some social security benefits that will help. Very occasionally the NHS will pay for care. You may need to unpick some complex issues depending on whether the support you are receiving is classed as 'nursing' or 'social' care. There are organisations that will help you to appeal against decisions if you are not happy. You need to find out under what circumstances the value of the person's house will or will not be taken into account and whether there will be a charge on its value to cover the fees. Age UK and Alzheimer's organisations will be able to help you with this. It used to be that in England and Wales local authorities could charge a husband, wife or civil partner, but that law was repealed in 2009.

The funding situation is so important and changeable that you must not rely on any information in a book or printed leaflet.

Find out directly what the situation is now from a reputable advisory organisation. A solicitor or the Citizens Advice Bureau may be able to help. Useful names are given at the end of the book. Not least, you need to be clear what is included in the fees that are being paid in the home and what is extra, such as laundry or outings.

Choosing the right place

It is essential to visit and see for yourself. Only if this is completely impossible should you delegate the job to a trusted friend or other family member. You can speak to a GP and ask local people about what they have experienced. Call associations such as Independent Age and the Relatives and Residents Association or Carers Direct (details at end of the book). Some solicitors offer a private 'social work' service to private clients.

I was on a one-year placement in New Zealand when my mother's dementia got so bad that she could not stay at home any longer. Her solicitor arranged for an experienced staff member to accompany her to visit a couple of recommended care homes and they negotiated a place, then helped to sell the house contents and put the house on the market. They kept up the visiting until I returned. (Caroline, daughter of woman with dementia)

The quality and standards of care provision in care homes are monitored and inspected by regulators in each of the four UK countries. Through them you can access reports online about the last inspection that took place and what the outcomes were. You can get this information from the Care Quality Commission in England, the Care Inspectorate in Scotland, the Care and Social Services Inspectorate in Wales or the Northern Ireland Regulation and Quality Improvement Authority.

Residents in care homes have rights. The following relates to England:

The Care Quality Commission (CQC) is the regulator of health and social care in England, whether it's provided by the NHS, local authorities, private companies or voluntary organisations.

Under existing rules, independent healthcare and adult social services should be registered with the CQC. NHS providers, such as hospitals and ambulance services, must also be registered. Registration of organisations reassures the public when they receive a care service or treatment. It also enables the CQC to check that organisations are continuing to meet CQC standards.

The standards set out the quality of care and facilities that you should expect from a care provider. As a resident in a care home, you should expect:

- *The right to be treated politely and with dignity.*
- *The right to privacy for yourself, and your relatives and friends when they visit.*
- *The right to deal with your own finances and spend your money how you choose.*
- *The right to eat food that's prepared in line with your faith and to worship when and where you want to.*
- *The right to choose the food that you eat, and to be given the time and space to relax and enjoy your meal.*
- *The right to choose when you get up in the mornings and go to bed at night.*
- *The right to complain if you're unhappy with your care.*

The National Minimum Standards for care homes are outlined on the CQC website.

These standards are not enforceable by law, but the CQC can enforce

fines, public warnings or close or suspend a service if they believe that
people's basic rights or safety are at risk. Organisations that are closed
or suspended are given the chance to meet the safety requirements and
resume their service. (www.nhs.uk/CarersDirect/guide/practicalsup-
port/Pages/Carehomes.aspx)

You may not want to imagine potential problems, but it is worth
getting confirmation of what will happen if the resident's condition deteriorates. Find out how much notice is given if they are
required to leave and how much notice you have to give if you
want to take them somewhere else. There is a difference between
what residential and nursing homes are prepared to do. Residential homes provide help with washing, dressing and medication,
going to the toilet, bathing and eating. Some have specialist training in dementia care. Nursing homes have a qualified nurse on
duty twenty-four hours a day and the care they provide is not just
about dementia but also other illnesses and disabilities. Not all
care homes are suitable for dementia and some are intolerant of
a number of the behavioural disturbances that may come with
dementia. Research shows that difficult behaviour is frequently
caused by the behaviour of the care workers and the design of
the home, so it is galling if this has caused the problem that the
home is not prepared to tolerate. But you still need a plan for
such a situation.

If the local authority is arranging for the admission and
there is more than one suitable home, the person has the right
to choose. A care home is suitable if it can meet the needs of
the person, the cost is right for the local authority and there is
an available place. The home must also be willing. You can 'top
up' if you have the resources and want something more than the
council is prepared to pay, but if you do this you need to be fairly
confident that there will be enough money to fund this going

forward. Moving to another home or a less pleasing room within a home is disturbing for a resident with dementia. If the worst happens and you feel that the money is running out, you need to talk to social services as early as possible to get the resident assessed again to see if they are able to help.

Once the person has taken up residence

Everyone said what a relief it must be for me when Mum went in the home, but it was just a different sort of stress. I could not believe that they would look after her properly, or understand her little ways. I cried myself to sleep every night. (H.L., daughter)

A good care home will appreciate it if you take an active role when you come to visit. What do you want to do? Take your mum for a bath or a stroll outside. Help go through her wardrobe sorting out minor repairs or items that need to be replaced. Sew tapes in her clothes and talk to her and sing. Have your supper with her in her room.

I did not like the way they did her hair, all brushed back in a band. She didn't even look like my mum any more. (H.L., daughter)

You can tell the home what you want. Provide a photograph of how she has always worn her hair. Talk to the hairdresser and her key worker. They should be glad to make a relationship with you. You can advise and ask for change.

The perfect care home

It has been described as being like a fine hotel with good house-keeping, a great restaurant and superior entertainment. Anyone who has to stay in hotels a lot will tell you that the charm soon wears off. You start to long for a place that feels like home, where you can do what you want. You wouldn't have to rush down for breakfast in case the buffet is closed. You wouldn't have to dress up. You could invite your friends round, or keep your dog with you, and you could stick things on the walls and make changes in your own space. You sometimes might not want to go to the dining room but just have beans on toast in front of the TV. Anyone who has to stay in hotels will tell you that the entertainment is for the lowest common denominator of the guests, and that's not you. The perfect care home is different for each of us. One person might like to socialise, while another might prefer to be alone. One might be glad to watch sport on TV all day, while another might need the peace and quiet of a garden. One might want to rest and another to be busy. The perfect care home for each of us is the one that allows us to do what we want.

And what about the end? I want to die with dignity if I can. I don't want to make a fuss or cause trouble. Please don't haul me about and drag me into and out of baths and talk about me as if I'm not there. Don't make me go to hospital right at the end if you can keep me comfortable in the home. But before all that happens, can we just try to have a little fun and laughter? I will if you will.

Chapter 15

Advice on complaints and sample letter

I write this chapter with a heavy heart. In one of my jobs, when I was the director of nursing of a large NHS Trust, I was responsible for handling every single formal complaint that came to us. I know that staff, including doctors and nurses, handled a lot of complaints informally.

This man was really angry about the way he found his mother in bed. She'd been incontinent and the sheets were wet and cold. We sorted her out as quickly as we could and I took him to one side to apologise. I told him that we really let ourselves down that day and that we understand how awful that must have been for her, and for him to discover it. I said there was no excuse, because although we were really busy, it should never have got to that. I was really, really sorry. The next day he brought me some flowers for the ward, and said he was sorry that he had complained because he knew we were so busy and he was really grateful for the way we care for her. I was a bit concerned in case he now felt he had to be nice to us, in case we took out our resentment on his mum. But actually, I really believe he was just relieved that he could say his piece and we listened and apologised and acted on it. (Ward sister)

The complaints that came to me were the ones where the staff had failed to satisfy the person, or where the person felt there was no point in talking to the staff. Some of those people were very,

very angry. They wrote or phoned and it was my job, along with a really small team of two part-time people, to acknowledge and respond quickly, and investigate if it was something complicated.

The longer we took to answer and respond, the angrier the people would be. We reduced the response time so much that we ended up phoning people on the day that their letters arrived. Often they were surprised to get such open, honest and fast interaction. They could explain the problem in their own words on the phone, and be given reassurance and some early answers. In certain cases they were satisfied at that stage, now that they knew what had happened and had got the irritation out.

A man wrote to complain about the hospital parking. I rang him back at once to talk to him, thinking I would explain about the new building work. I asked him to tell me the whole story. His dad had a blood test and was told to come to the hospital to get the result. The son and his wife have only one car and a small child, so he had to take a day off work to allow him to use the car to drive his dad to the hospital as well as take the child to nursery. When he got to the hospital, early, he drove round for half an hour to find a space. When he got his dad to the clinic, dead on time, he found that the person in front had not attended, and that the doctor already had left, assuming that he would not attend either.

I don't think the problem was the parking, really. The problem was the stupidity of having to attend hospital to get the result of a blood test, and the rule that only the doctor could impart it, and that the doctor felt able to walk away early from the clinic. So I rang the clinic, got the man's test result and gave it to him over the phone. I could not have fixed it if I did not have that authority and did not make that phone call. He withdrew his complaint. (Clinic manager)

The National Health Service in the UK is the world's largest publicly funded health service. It often takes a beating in the press and is used as a political football, but because it employs over one and a half million people and deals with over a million patients every thirty-six hours you can expect that some things will go wrong. That said, some areas of its work are really worrying, in particular the culture of care for older people and those with dementia. Dementia has been with us since long before the creation of the NHS, but it is only recently that it has come to the fore as a priority area of treatment. So you should not expect perfection, and should have a good idea of what to do if it falls short for you.

One problem with complaining is that the complaints system is not very intelligent, agile or flexible, and the overwhelming bureaucracy makes it seem defensive and secretive. There is an interesting contrast these days between people who are afraid to complain in case retribution is handed out to them and people who, once they start to complain, allow their grievance to take over their whole life. Those who get into that state have often been incensed as a result of the problems of the complaints process, which is unfortunately designed to be more about redress than mediation. Mediation would be better.

However, we are in a position where you may have to complain using the current complaints processes to get what you want. It is better in the first place to be able to get what you want through a health and social care system that works well helped by having knowledge of how to make the system work.

Social work assessments, for example, can be a nightmare and having some information in advance on what words and expressions will trigger the response you want is a good idea. What is provided from social services varies by region, so it is important to know how to find out what is available in your own part of the country. Even the variation in the names of the different departments and officials can be disconcerting. You need to understand that sometimes the person you are speaking to may know less about dementia and the local system than you do, so it is helpful to know how to negotiate past that without setting yourself up as a 'vexatious' client. At times you may have to complain. In order to get what you want, you may have to ask repeatedly for things. On the other hand, if you don't accept services as they are, at the pace they are provided, you may start to be regarded as a pest. All organisations have vexatious complainant policies.

The London Borough of X aims to provide high-quality services to all of our customers ... In those cases where our customers, staff or the council as a whole suffer adversely from persons making repeated, frivolous or persistent complaints or who do so in a threatening, abusive or difficult way our Persistent and Vexatious Complainants Policy will be applied ... For the purposes of this policy we have adopted the Local Government Ombudsman's (LGO) definition of 'unreasonable persistent complaints' and 'unreasonable complainant behaviour'. (Extract from a council complaints process)

It all depends on how you decide what is 'reasonable'. Advice on how to complain about a range of services depends on what the issue is. In general, it is important to:

- understand the problem;
- know the system and key people in it;
- be known to them as a usually positive client;
- use high-impact communication;
- persevere.

And I usually say you also need to be lucky ...

To help with your communications, look at the sample letter in this chapter and at the organisations listed at the end of the book.

People are ambivalent about the NHS. On the one hand, they are sentimental about it, and think of the people working there as heroes, but on the other they are prepared to believe it is falling to bits, even if we don't have direct or personal local evidence.

I know it badly needs to change. We hear about terrible things in the NHS all the time, but it's always very, very good here. We could not ask for more. (John, 83)

Even those who work within the NHS have a culture of ambivalence about their relationship with it.

Sometimes people would say, 'I didn't really want the complaint to go this far.' It was remarkable how many complainants had mentioned that they were disappointed (for example, when they waited a long time for a clinic) and our own doctors and nurses had said, 'You need to complain to the managers and write to your MP about this.' It was as if the only way the staff could bring their own concern about the service forward was by using the patients' families as cannon fodder. Then they just got on with their lives as if they had no responsibility for the management of expectations. If they were better organised themselves the waits would be shorter. And I don't want to gag them from speaking in public, but why didn't they tell me directly? It's as if they want to give a public impression that we are falling apart. (Trust chief executive)

There is a difference between complaining about a service that has been given and challenging a decision that the health and social care system has made about your entitlement to care.

Following a critical report from the ombudsman in 2003, the NHS in England had to identify thousands of individuals who had been denied continuing care and reimburse care costs sometimes going back as far as 1996. There are solicitors who make a living out of challenging NHS continuing-care decisions in

England. Because the process for questioning these decisions is complex, you may decide that you want professional help if you don't like the outcome. The assessor may have misunderstood some of the issues, or they may not have counted up some of the needs that are already being met. They are supposed to include them – they don't cease to exist just because someone else has addressed them. The solicitor will be better able to help you if you have detailed records telling the true story of what help is needed. You should keep a diary if you can. In the end you can go to the Health Service Ombudsman. In Scotland the decision can be reviewed by the NHS Board and you can use the NHS complaints procedure and eventually the Scottish Public Services Ombudsman.

This is quite different from the situation where you believe that an act or omission by someone in the health and social care system has caused you harm, such as when a doctor or dentist may be accused of clinical negligence. The General Medical Council deals with the most serious complaints about doctors, and the Nursing and Midwifery Council about nurses. There are a number of other organisations that might help and these differ across the four countries of the UK. In England there is Healthwatch (www.healthwatch.co.uk). In Scotland you can find the Health Rights Information Scotland (www.hris.org.uk) and the Patient Advice and Support Service (www.patientadvicescotland.org.uk). Northern Ireland has the Patient and Client Council (www.patientclientcouncil.hscni.net) and Wales has the Community Health Councils and Putting Things Right (www.wales.nhs.uk). In each case there is also the ombudsman for each country (details at the end of the book).

The culture of the system

The process of assessment for dementia was described in Chapter 2, and the health care workers involved should have done this in an energetic and interactive way that included the family as well as the person with dementia. What happens from the beginning of your journey should be a matter of negotiation. Yet you may sometimes feel that the health and social care professionals have all the power and that you wait on them for their attention and the resources that they will give you. The very best systems will give power to those they are helping, and everyone can share responsibility for what happens. It is worth being aware that some of the people in the system themselves do not feel powerful. Why else would they ask patients to intercede on their behalf with the management through the complaints system?

The statistics suggested that most complaints are about care of older people and a lot are about how a few of the consultants communicate. It was suggested to me that they don't know how to communicate. My view is that they communicate loud and clear and all too well. But they communicate the wrong message: e.g. that they are tired, and impatient, and angry, and dismissive. (NHS complaints officer)

People with dementia do not wish to be patronised, and they are not deaf or insensitive. In some ways they are more sensitive than the rest of us, who can be blinded by words so that we miss the non-verbal communications. It is known that health and social care workers do not have a range of registers that they can vary according to their audience. It might be mistaken for egalitarianism to address everyone with the same cheery 'mate' or some other endearment. In the NHS you should expect more, but you have to decide what you are going to do about it if you don't get it. It would be good if all staff had a variety of ways of addressing people, and were nice and discreet. Whether that happens or not depends, according to the research, on the characteristics of the person in charge of the clinical area.

I was in the corridor outside the ward and I heard someone roar, 'DOES HE HAVE A CATHETER?' I had a vision of someone going off to check under the bedclothes to see if some poor man had a rubber tube coming out of his penis. Or maybe not yet, because moments later the nurse had to roar it out again. I entered the ward and the shouter, who turned out to be the man in charge, gave me a wide smile and cheerful, 'Good morning.' I can only guess what the patients thought of that. (Hospital visitor)

You will find that people do not speak to you or the person with dementia as you would wish. You will also find that you are not given enough information. At the same time as not telling you what you need to know, they sometimes give you more information than you need to know about stuff you do not need to know.

The nurse was in the house for fifteen minutes, during which she spoke about her overtime, colleagues off sick, the cutbacks, the chance of early retirement, how the NHS was better in the old days, how her car was unreliable and people would die as a result of the closure of the old wing of the hospital, she expected. She failed to tell Fred how to change the catheter bag or maintain his hygiene or prevent a urine infection. (Niece, 58)

Congratulations and complaints

The best letter to be able to send to the health and social care system is one where you are saying thank you for a job well done, and there are lots of times when you will be able to send such a letter. We generally expect the system to work, and we walk away happy when it does, without necessarily saying much. If you're not happy you have a right to complain, but it's important to first think what it is you want to achieve. It could be that you only want an apology or an explanation, but you might be looking for some form of redress. Once you start any legal action, the complaints system is closed to you. You may wonder how to go about complaining. The cheerful instruction from Northern Ireland is that you can complain 'in the way that best suits you'. The complaints system for health and social care is very similar. You can find out about your local authority at www.gov.uk/find-your-local-council.

It is very important to raise any issues as soon as possible with the staff with whom you have direct contact, and if they can't answer you as you'd wish you need to ask for their manager or supervisor, and eventually the chief executive of the organisation or the complaints team if they have one. Please don't be afraid that you'll receive worse treatment as a result of the complaint. That would not be a rational response of the system. If you want things to be better you should not miss your chance of telling someone, and in what way you think it could be better. In general there is a time limit of twelve months after the event, unless you've got a good reason for not knowing you had a concern.

Every NHS organisation, social work department and care home has a complaints procedure. It should be easy to find on their website, on signs in their premises, or by asking a member of staff. In many places a copy of the procedure will be given to you even if you don't ask for it. The NHS undergoes major changes in core structure at regular intervals, particularly in England though it's true to an extent for some of the rest of the UK NHS; however, the complaints process remains relatively stable. There are specific rights outlined in each of the four countries, but in general they all offer that:

- Your complaint will be dealt with efficiently, properly and within a certain period of time.
- You'll know the outcome.
- You have somewhere to go (an ombudsman) if you're not happy with the way the complaint was handled.
- You can make a request for a judicial review if you think what happened was unlawful.
- You can be compensated if you've been harmed.

In England you need to complain to a local organisation that was set up in 2013 called your Clinical Commissioning Group, or you can contact NHS England (England.contactus@nhs.net).

You can get help from:

- PALS (Patient Advice and Liaison Service) in your local hospital;
- NHS Complaints Independent Advocacy Service (arrangements vary between each local authority area);
- Citizens Advice Bureau.

In Wales, if the Health Board does not satisfy you or follow its own correct procedure you can contact the Public Services Ombudsman for Wales. Your local Community Health Council can help you with your complaints through their free independent complaints advocacy service. They can offer support by:

- giving you advice;
- explaining your options;
- informing you of your rights;
- assisting you with correspondence;
- supporting you in meetings;
- voicing your concerns;

● accessing your health records.

In Scotland there is an organisation called PASS (Patient Advice and Support Service) provided through the Citizens Advice Bureau. As with the Community Health Council in Wales, it offers practical help in making a complaint, including writing letters, making phone calls and supporting you in preparing for and attending meetings. The advice guide is clearly aimed at linking your complaint with what you ought to expect if you have a range of conditions, but dementia is not one of them at the time of writing.

The difference in Northern Ireland is that health and social care services are integrated already. There are plans for this in Scotland. For complaints in Northern Ireland, the General Medical Council website (www.gmc-uk.org) advises:

You should try to provide details of:

● how to contact you;

● who or what you are complaining about;

● where and when the event that caused your complaint happened; and,

● if possible, what you would like to be done to address your complaint.

Sample letter of complaint

The following letter will give you an idea of how to complain. You need to include your full address and phone numbers. If you'd be happy to receive emails that is sometimes helpful for speeding things up. Use the information on the organisation's website to be sure that you are sending your letter to the right person, otherwise it will go round and round the system and get lost. In general, the more senior the person you write to the better.

Make sure you have the name of the person affected correct. You want to use the name and if possible the numbers that they are known by, and details of when the contact was: for example, dates of admission to the care home, or dates of visits by the care staff.

It is good to have a clear idea of what you are complaining about. It is always sensible to ask questions, because that shapes the answer you get. There is no need to use emotional language in your first communication. Just stick to the facts to begin with, although you should make it clear that you are puzzled and disappointed not to have received the right treatment. Remember to keep copies of everything and note your date of posting the letter.

It is a shame to have to strike a discordant note when so many people work very hard to make a system work. Sometimes, however, the system just needs a bit of encouragement to improve.

---

24 Acacia Gardens	Tel. 0123 456 7890
Oldfield	Mobile 07901 234567
Grantchester	
EH15 3BB	Email bloggs@acacia.net

29 June 2014

Dear Mr Smith

Patient number 7966 – James Blogg –
Date of Birth 29/6/35

I am writing to you about my father, James Blogg, who was a

patient in your hospital on Ward 10 from 1 to 14 May. I have power of attorney for him and his permission to discuss these issues with you.

I made a complaint to the nurse in charge of the ward on 3 May, 5 May, 12 May and 14 May with no satisfactory conclusion. The nurse was Fred Green on 3 May and Mary Brown on the other dates.

Your website states that you will do your best to consult a next of kin or advocate about any serious treatment that you need to give.

On four separate occasions I discovered my father had been visited by doctors and assumed to agree to treatments and then his discharge without any reference to me.

I had concerns about the amount he had to eat and drink during his admission. He lost so much weight and whenever I visited his water jug was almost always out of reach.

I would like you to investigate the understanding that your staff have of your own complaints processes, your procedures on consent and capability, and all issues concerning people with dementia.

I need to be confident that he'll be treated properly if he ever returns to your hospital. Please tell me what training the staff have had on these matters. Did they know that he has dementia and how was that reflected in his care? How was his weight and fluid intake recorded?

Please carry out a full investigation into my concerns and provide a full response within your stated NHS complaints procedure and timescales.

Yours sincerely
Mary Blogg

Postscript

Since the first edition of this book was published the research on dementia has moved on and there have been a number of huge disappointments for people affected by dementia. It is probably ten years since I first heard at a dementia research conference about the need for a 'paradigm shift' in research about dementia – and sadly, that is still the case. What does that mean? It means that all the things we used to think about how to cure dementia need to be considered in a completely different way.

Firstly, we need to consider how useful it is to have an 'umbrella' term for dementia, bearing in mind how many different disease conditions cause dementia. All those different diseases require different cures, even if the effects they have on people are similar. Then, of course, we may remember that we needed the umbrella term only because often we have no idea which disease is causing the cluster of symptoms and the evidence of brain failure. It is rare to find someone with only Alzheimer's or only vascular disease and people often have a mix, not to mention the hundreds of other diseases. And then there is the strange fact that we find people who have Alzheimer's disease changes very evidently in their brain at post mortem, who never exhibited signs of dementia in their behaviour while they were alive. Why do only some people with Alzheimer's disease get dementia? And who are the small group of people diagnosed with dementia who have survived and are living well for a decade or more? Is this just missed or a mistaken diagnosis? Or something quite odd and different – a functional neurological disorder? We need to be clearer about what we mean by 'dementia'.

Secondly, when politicians set a political goal of finding a cure within a certain time span, they are ignoring the science. Time and again pharmaceutical companies have abandoned trials of medication that they hoped would modify Alzheimer's disease. Politicians have come and gone, in the life time of this little book, promising that a cure would be found by a certain date, and it's clear that they didn't know what they were talking about. False hope continues to be given by media reports that exaggerate the effects of small trials, and anyone who questions this misrepresentation is thought of as damaging morale. It's a sort of treachery in the dementia community to tell the truth. We need to resist this pressure and focus more on helping people now who are affected by dementia in the present, rather than asking them to imagine that there is a cure round the corner for them. Implementing what we already know would be a good start. Let's be practical.

And finally, in developed countries, the number of people with age-related dementia is not increasing at the rate we expected. Prevalence of dementia is falling. There are strange relationships between things like childhood trauma or social isolation that seem related to dementia, but we have no clear idea why. The newly named condition Limbic-predominant Age-related TDP-43 Encephalopathy (LATE) is being called as important as Alzheimer's disease in people over the age of 80 in the explanation of dementia. LATE is something that we will hear more of in the coming years.

So what does this mean if you are affected now, or want to avoid being affected in future? The answer is this. If you are lucky enough to grow old, you will have many things that contribute to your health or illness. This includes your genes, and having the right parents. It includes other illness that you may manage carefully, like diabetes. There will be lifestyle-related factors that you may control such as your weight and fitness, your visceral body fat and the size of your muscles, and the amount of time you have spent developing your brain. It will be luck, such as whether you suffered childhood trauma, a head injury, or have a personality that makes you predisposed to loneliness. Hopefully this book will have given you some sense of how to manage these elements, and what the best practice is for tending to your ongoing health.

In 2019, the World Health Organization produced guidelines on dementia that echo the advice in this book. There are twelve recommendations or areas that we need to attend to, and they are, at this time, the last word on the subject. All of these are areas that national governments can prioritise, but each of us can attend to them in our own lives, to stay as well as possible for as long as possible. They fall under headings of:

- Physical activity
- Tobacco cessation
- Nutritional interventions
- Interventions for alcohol-use disorders
- Cognitive interventions
- Social activity
- Weight management
- Management of high blood pressure
- Management of diabetes
- Management of cholesterol

- Management of depression
- Management of hearing loss.

  www.who.int/mental_health/neurology/dementia/guidelines _risk_reduction/en/

Dementia is a feminist issue

In 2015, with the support of the Dementia Services Development Trust, I conducted a survey to determine how thinking about dementia had changed over the previous twenty-five years. We had seen media reports that people today are more afraid of dementia than cancer, and we wanted to know if that was true. Did people believe, as has been reported, that health and social care workers do not provide care based on research evidence? What plans did people think they needed to make for their loved one? Nearly 3,000 people completed the survey. Although we tried very hard to get both men and women to complete the survey, men were much less likely to do so. The most remarkable finding was that the men who did complete the survey differed radically from the women in how they think about dementia:

- Although most people know that dementia is caused by an underlying disease, men are twice as likely as women to regard dementia as part of normal ageing.
- Men are also more likely than women to believe that people with dementia can be cured.
- More men than women believe that drugs are or will be the answer.
- Men seem to have greater confidence than women that how patients with dementia are treated in hospitals is based on research.

- More men than women believe that you and your family should contribute to care, either by providing it or by paying for it.
- When asked, men had more confidence than women that better awareness in the community would help with dementia, but women had a stronger belief that improving the knowledge of care staff is needed.
- Women are much more aware of the dangers of a hospital admission than men are.
- More women than men have a negative experience of being listened to by the health care system.
- More women than men fear dementia and say they'd rather die than be affected by it.
- More women than men responded positively to the idea of voluntary euthanasia.

Looking at the raw data, we wondered whether this difference between genders was a modern phenomenon. And how much had the way people regard dementia changed, even in our own professional lifetimes and in the history of the Dementia Services Development Trust?

In the 1970s, just before the Trust was created, institutional care for people with dementia was improving but still included some dreadful practices. Health care workers performed their tasks as fast as possible so that they could sit down for a cup of tea and a cigarette. To speed up the bathing routine, for example, patients would be stripped naked in front of each other in a production line.

When I was a nursing student in a large psychiatric hospital in the 1980s, more enlightened textbooks suggested that curtains be hung between the bathtubs in the bathroom so that patients could not see each other but the nurse could still supervise them all. I saw people tied to the toilet pan so that they wouldn't leave the bathroom while staff fetched other patients. Even in those days, any staff or students who complained about this sort of humiliation would be labelled as squeamish and unsuitable for nursing work with people who had dementia. A good nurse was someone who could 'bathe and toilet' a lot of people quickly. That task was made easier by heaps of communal apparel, which allowed nursing staff to dress people in whatever was at hand, including dresses for women with slit openings at the back to make it easier for staff to manhandle them in the toilet. People who could still walk were put in wheelchairs and hurled along corridors because they did not move fast enough for the staff. Eventually they would lose the power to walk unaided purely because they were not allowed to take time to continue doing things for themselves. The situation is much better now, but the horror of institutional care in former times still taints how we think about dementia today.

Surveys make most sense if you compare them with a baseline, and unfortunately, there is no proper baseline for how people in general used to think about dementia. We know that people twenty to thirty years ago did not speak much about dementia, and a lot of what was said was wrong. In addition, because a lot of what has been written in the past was written by men, it is hard to make a gendered analysis of what people were thinking.

It is said that before the rise of Victorian institutions, 'the family' used to take care of old people. What caused this norm to change from home care to institutional care? I believe that because family care is usually done by women, the increased opportunities for women in the workplace may have been a key factor in the creation of institutions. Is it more cost effective for your daughter to stay at home and look after you or for her to go out to work? Which of these two options can the family best afford? As more women entered the workplace and obtained higher-paying jobs, and as family size decreased, institutions came into their own.

Today, however, most people with dementia are living in their own homes, even if they have no family. As the cost of care homes rises, will women again in future forgo opportunities to work or study because they need to care for their frail older parents? And how does all this affect the way people think about dementia?

The preponderance of women looking after people with dementia suggests that women have a greater reason to take an interest in old age, frailty and dementia than men. In the University of Stirling Dementia Centre funded by the Dementia Trust, male employees – including academics, managers and others – had never been more than 10 per cent of the staff. Later we began to examine the gender balance of the people who create government policies on dementia.

A global research review had already been undertaken by Alzheimer's Disease International in 2015. The purpose of that report was to understand the dementia-related issues affecting women internationally. The report looked at women living with dementia, women caring for people with dementia in a professional role, and women undertaking an informal caregiving role for someone with dementia. The report also looked at factors affecting women in low- and middle-income countries, at family structures and kinship, and at the effect of migration on women.

The key findings of this report are startling. The prevalence of dementia is higher in women, and they live with more severe symptoms. They are also more likely to be informal carers or even professional carers. The report noted that there is very little research on the gender issues in dementia.

Over 60 per cent of people with dementia are female. This is partly because women live longer and dementia is related to age.

But that is not all. As this book has explained, dementia is not a disease but the symptom of any of a range of diseases, the commonest of which is Alzheimer's. In contrast to other diseases, the severity of the symptoms is not always directly related to the severity of the underlying disease. Symptoms are made worse by depression, loneliness, poor diet and lack of exercise – problems that are worse for anyone who has fewer resources.

The current generation of older women – particularly married women – have often depended on a man's occupational pension in old age because these women had mainly worked at home performing domestic and caregiving tasks. Until relatively recent times, if a man and a woman divorced, the woman's unwaged contribution to the family resources would probably not be compensated, leaving her in poverty in old age even if her husband was still alive. Even today, the death of a husband or partner can leave a woman who has never participated in the workforce in difficult financial circumstances. The same is true for a man who loses his partner, but he is more likely to have earned and saved more and is more likely to have benefited from an occupational pension. So in general, older women are likely to be less well off than men, and being poor makes some of the things that would reduce dementia symptoms simply unaffordable. The 2016 change in UK pension age for women has left a cohort of women born in the 1950s considerably worse off than they expected.

Research also shows other ways in which women can be disproportionately affected by dementia and old-age frailty.

For example, when an older woman has a husband with dementia she often has the life skills to care for him, so he is more likely to end his days in reasonable comfort at home, especially as she is probably a little bit younger than he is. When an older woman has dementia, the reverse is often true – her husband may not have the skills to care for her, so she is more likely to end her days not in comfort and not at home, especially since he is probably a bit older than she is – which is another reason why a disproportionate number of residents in care homes are women.

Men may be caregivers for their elderly parents, but most of this work falls on daughters, granddaughters and nieces. And this gender disparity is not just seen in the home. Workers in dementia care, who are mainly women, earn low wages and are often not held in high esteem, which is reflected in their working conditions.

Research shows that stress in midlife is related to dementia in later life, and in many cases women's lives in the last century have been more stressful than men's because of lower pay and less financial security in old age, less protection against sex discrimination and violence, and the hazards of childbirth, among other things. Women at the height of their professional careers were also more likely to be doing the largest share of childcare, housework and looking after elderly relatives. Older women have often experienced stresses in their lives that we will never know about. How recently did unmarried women have their children ripped away from them for adoption or deportation in an atmosphere of violence and disgrace? What other painful and stressful secrets might they carry related to previous miscarriages or abortions that could not be discussed?

These statements should not be misinterpreted as a diatribe from someone who does not like men and refuses to recognise their contribution to care work, which can be as heroic as any woman's. But the statistics do not lie. We need to celebrate the lives of the older women we care for now that they are in their eighties and nineties. These women were the pioneers who did without many of the benefits that they subsequently won for us – such as maternity leave and allowances, equal rights at work, laws that work against violence and rape, recognition of the need for education for girls, decent sanitary products, washing machines and disposable nappies.

The difference in how men and women regard euthanasia needs to be explored more carefully. It is not clear whether those who would rather die are afraid of being humiliated and badly cared for or whether they would prefer to avoid the cost of that care so that they can leave a legacy for their children. It could also be connected to the fact that women have less confidence in the possibility of a scientific cure. The fact that men may have more confidence that science will find a cure for dementia is not in itself a bad thing unless it distracts us from the need to provide care and support now, to the women (and men) who are most affected by this sometimes cruel affliction.

Although bad things still happen in a care setting, the situation in general is much better now than it was in the early 1980s. The ideal of support at home followed, if needed, by a move to a homelike setting is a reality for many people. Good meals, exercise, entertainment, company, privacy, dignity – all of these are expected now. But I wanted to know whether that has made a difference in how people think about dementia. It is always frustrating that every research report ends by saying, 'More research is needed.' But in this case it is all too true.

Those people and organisations that are shaping policy about dementia need to defend themselves against a possible accusation that men are making policy decisions about what is essentially a women's issue. A quick glance at the executives of a number of elected bodies, advocacy organisations and research establishments reflects the current prevalence of men at the top in business and society. This must change in all walks of life, but change in organisations that are shaping policy about dementia is urgent in light of what we are learning about the difference in attitudes towards dementia between men and women. The voices of women caregivers and women with dementia must be heard and must have a role in shaping policy.

Resources and helpful organisations

Updates to this book are on www.juneandrews.net, and you can make comments or ask for further information there.

WHO guidelines on risk reduction of cognitive decline and dementia www.who.int/mental_health/neurology/dementia/risk_reduction_gdg_meeting/en/

Key resources

The following are available from Amazon:

- June Andrews and Allan House, *10 Helpful Hints for Carers: Practical Solutions for Carers Living with People with Dementia*
- Dementia Services Development Centre, *10 Helpful Hints for Dementia Design at Home: Practical Design Solutions for Carers Living at Home with Someone Who Has Dementia*
- June Andrews, *Care Homes: The One-Stop Guide: When, Why and How to Choose a Care Home* (Profile Books, 2020)

Children's books about dementia

- Jessica Shepherd, *Grandma*: a grandmother becomes increasingly forgetful and moves into a home

- Ruth Eastham, *The Memory Cage*: a boy from Bosnia tries to get his grandad to keep his memories, but the memories are painful because of war
- Irene Mackay, *The Forgetful Elephant*: a story of how a little elephant copes when her grandfather starts to forget her.
- David Walliams, *Grandpa's Great Escape*: a funny story of how Grampa escapes from his care home away from an evil matron.

Life-story work

Life-story work is described on YouTube (www.youtube.com/watch?v=5JjCwoJLoXM), and information about how to make and use a Life Story book can be found at www.dementiauk.org/wp-content/uploads/2017/03/Lifestory-.compressed.pdf.

Useful organisations

Action on Elder Abuse (all countries)
Charity in the UK working exclusively on this issue, providing knowledge, expertise and support to thousands of people every year
080 8808 8141
www.elderabuse.org.uk

Age Cymru
Information for people in later life, through its advice line, publications and website
0800 022 3444
www.agecymru.org.uk

Age NI
Information for people in later life, through its advice line, publications and website

0808 808 7575

www.ageni.org

Age Scotland

Information for people in later life, through its advice line, publications and website

0800 124 4222

www.agescotland.org.uk

Age UK (for England)

Information for people in later life, through its advice line, publications and website

0800 169 6565 (lines open seven days a week, 8 a.m.–7 p.m.)

www.ageuk.org.uk

Alzheimer Scotland

160 Dundee Street

Edinburgh EH11 1DQ

0131 243 1453

Email: info@alzscot.org

www.alzscot.org

Alzheimer's Research UK

(formerly Alzheimer's Research Trust)

3 Riverside

Granta Park

Cambridge CB21 6AD

0300 111 5555

Email: enquiries@alzheimersresearchuk.org

www.alzheimersresearchuk.org

Alzheimer's Society

Legal and welfare helpline, plus information on legal and welfare issues

0845 300 0336
www.alzheimers.org.uk

Alzheimer's Society Northern Ireland

30 Skegoneill Street
Belfast BT15 3JL
Helpline: 0300 222 1122
Switchboard: 028 9066 4100
Email: nir@alzheimers.org.uk
www.alzheimers.org.uk/about-us/northern-ireland

Care and Social Services Inspectorate Wales (CSSIW)

0300 7900 126
www.careinspectorate.wales

Carers Direct

*Ask questions using webchat; helpline Monday to Friday, 9 a.m.–8
p.m. and weekends 11 a.m.–4 p.m. Also you can email via NHS
Choices*
0300 123 1053

Carers NI (Northern Ireland)

028 9043 9843
www.carersuk.org

Carers Trust Charity

Supporting carers
0300 772 9600
www.carers.org

Carers UK (includes Carers Scotland and Carers Wales)

0808 808 7777
www.carersuk.org

Care Quality Commission in England (CQC)

Registration and inspection of care homes in England
03000 616161
www.cqc.org.uk

Chartered Society of Physiotherapy

The professional, educational and trade union body for chartered physiotherapists, physiotherapy students and assistants. Provides contact details of private physiotherapists in your area
14 Bedford Row
London WC1R 4ED
020 7306 6666
Email: enquiries@csp.org.uk
www.csp.org.uk

Citizens Advice Bureau (CAB)

Your local CAB can provide information and advice in confidence or point you in the right direction. To find your nearest CAB look in the phone book, ask at your local library or look on the Citizens Advice website. Opening times vary
www.citizensadvice.org.uk

The College of Podiatry

The professional body and trade union for registered podiatrists. Provides patient information on common foot problems and details of private practice podiatrists
Quartz House
207 Providence Square
Mill Street
London SE1 2EW
020 7234 8620
www.cop.org.uk/

Crossroads Caring Scotland
Support for carers and their families in Scotland
www.crossroads-scotland.co.uk/

Gov.UK
Brilliant website for information
www.gov.uk

Independent Age
Advice and guidance for older people
0800 319 6789
www.independentage.org

The Lewy Body Society
Unity House, Westwood Park
Wigan WN3 4HE
01942 914000
www.lewybody.org/

NHS Direct
0845 4647/or simply: 111 (lines open 24 hours a day, seven days a week)
www.111.nhs.uk

NHS online information
www.nhs.uk

Office of Care and Protection (Northern Ireland)
www.nidirect.gov.uk/contacts/contacts-az/
office-care-and-protection

Office of the Public Guardian (England)
Archway Tower, 9 Junction Road, London N19 5SZ
Enduring power of attorney helpline: 0845 330 2963 (Monday to
Friday, 9 a.m.–5 p.m.)

Literature and application forms: 0845 330 2900 (Monday to
Friday, 9 a.m.–5 p.m.)
Email: custserv@guardianship.gov.uk
www.gov.uk/government/organisations/
office-of-the-public-guardian
SEE ALSO public guardian in **Scotland**
www.publicguardianscotland.gov.uk/

Parkinson's UK
215 Vauxhall Bridge Road
London SW1V 1EJ
020 7931 8080
www.parkinsons.org.uk

Relatives and Residents Association
020 7359 8136
www.relres.org

Royal College of Speech and Language Therapists
*The professional body for speech and language therapists and support
workers. Promotes excellence in practice and influences health,
education and social care policies*
2 White Hart Yard
London SE1 1NX
020 7378 1200
Email: info@rcslt.org
www.rcslt.org

Scottish Partnership for Palliative Care
*An umbrella and representative organisation which supports and
contributes to the development and strategic direction of palliative
care in Scotland*
CBC House, 24 Canning Street

Edinburgh EH3 8EG

0131 272 2735

Email: office@palliativecarescotland.org.uk

www.palliativecarescotland.org.uk

An ombudsman exists for each of the four administrations in the UK:

Local Government Ombudsman

PO Box 4771

Coventry CVB4 0EH

0300 061 0614

www.lgo.org.uk

Parliamentary and Health Service Ombudsman

Millbank Tower

Millbank

London SW1P 4QP

0345 015 4033

Email: phso.enquiries@ombudsman.org.uk

www.ombudsman.org.uk/

Public Services Ombudsman for Northern Ireland

Progressive House

33 Wellington Place

Belfast BT1 6HN

Freephone: 0800 343 424

Tel.: 028 9023 3821

www.nipso.org.uk

Public Services Ombudsman for Scotland

Bridgeside House

99 McDonald Road

Edinburgh EH7 4NS
0800 377 7330
www.spso.org.uk/

Public Services Ombudsman for Wales
1 Ffordd yr Hen Gae
Pencoed CF35 5LJ
0300 790 0203
www.ombudsman.wales

Acknowledgements

I want to thank Andrew Franklin, Louisa Dunnigan, Graeme Hall and the staff of Profile Books for encouragement, expertise and advice in putting the book together.

My own knowledge is enriched by many conversations with people diagnosed with dementia and their families, in particular Dr James McKillop who proofread the first edition, and I thank Sandra McDonald, Rev Nigel Robb, Dr Cesar Rodriguez and Trustees of the Dementia Services Development Trust for their advice and support with the text. All those who worked at the Dementia Services Development Centre at the University of Stirling have shaped my thinking.

Thanks are due to my husband Charles and daughter Charlotte who give me peace to write. I am also thankful for the support of members of my family and friends, including Mark Butler, Professor Allan House, Sonia Mangan and Maureen McGinn who read drafts and put up with my absence while I was writing.

In particular, I am grateful for the tireless support and encouragement of my sister Hazel McKay who read and commented on proofs. She's a saint.

Index

CENTRAL 18·11·2020